Parental Obligations and

T0251902

This book investigates what obligations a parent incurs by bringing a child into being. In other words, it shares with Mary Shelley—from whose *Frankenstein* the book's subtitle is derived—an interest in the duties of parents as creators, or, as the author writes, "qua procreators." Toward this end, the book develops accounts both of how parental obligations are acquired and what these obligations amount to. Its basic thesis is that parents, as procreators, have obligations regarding future children that put constraints on procreative liberty. Moreover, these obligations go beyond respecting a child's rights, in particular the oft-invoked child's right to an open future. The author brings the book's account of parental obligations to bear on the ethics of adoption, child support, gamete donation, surrogacy, and prenatal genetic enhancement. A final chapter examines the question of public responsibility for children and argues that it is much greater than typically acknowledged.

Bernard G. Prusak is Associate Professor of Philosophy and Director of the McGowan Center for Ethics and Social Responsibility at King's College in Wilkes-Barre, PA, USA.

Routledge Annals of Bioethics

Edited by Mark J. Cherry, St. Edward's University, USA and
Ana Smith Iltis, Wake Forest University, USA

Parental Obligations and Bioethics

The Duties of a Creator

Bernard G. Prusak

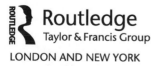

Routledge
Taylor & Francis Group

LONDON AND NEW YORK

First published 2013 by Routledge

2 Park Square, Milton Park, Abingdon, Oxon OX14 4RN
711 Third Avenue, New York, NY 10017, USA

*Routledge is an imprint of the Taylor & Francis Group,
an informa business*

First issued in paperback 2016

Copyright © 2013 Taylor & Francis

The right of Bernard G. Prusak to be identified as author of this work
has been asserted by him/her in accordance with sections 77 and 78 of
the Copyright, Designs and Patents Act 1988.

Library of Congress Cataloging-in-Publication Data

Prusak, Bernard G.
  Parental obligations and bioethics : the duties of a creator / by Bernard
  G. Prusak. — 1 [edition].
    pages cm. — (Routledge annals of bioethics ; 14)
  Includes bibliographical references and index.
 1. Bioethics.   2. Parenting—Moral and ethical aspects.
3. Child rearing—Moral and ethical aspects.   4. Sexual ethics.
I. Title.
  QH332.P78 2013
  174.2—dc23
  2013013957

ISBN: 978-0-415-70333-8 (hbk)
ISBN: 978-1-138-24530-3 (pbk)

Typeset in Sabon
by Apex CoVantage, LLC

For M.S.K., in gratitude, and in memory of my mother

Contents

Acknowledgments

Parts of this book are derived from material that first saw the light of day in rougher forms. I am grateful to the various publishers both for permission to reprint this material and for seeing value in my articles. I thank series editors Mark Cherry and Ana Smith Iltis for seeing value in this book.

Chapter 1 draws from and significantly recasts "What Are Parents For? Reproductive Ethics after the Non-Identity Problem," *Hastings Center Report* 40/2 (2010): 37–47. Chapter 2 draws from, corrects, and extends both "The Costs of Procreation," *Journal of Social Philosophy* 42/1 (2011): 61–75 and "Whither the 'Offices of Nature'? Kant and the Obligation to Love," *Proceedings of the American Catholic Philosophical Association* 83 (2009): 113–128. Chapter 3 draws from, and counters criticisms raised by, "Breaking the Bond: Abortion and the Grounds of Parental Obligations," *Social Theory and Practice* 37/2 (2011): 311–332. Chapter 5 is based on "Not Good Enough Parenting: What's Wrong with the Child's Right to an 'Open Future,'" *Social Theory and Practice* 34/2 (2008): 271–291. Finally, chapter 6 modifies "Paying for the Priceless Child," *Proceedings of the American Catholic Philosophical Association* 86 (2012).

The quotations from Job in chapters 1 and 2 are taken from the New Revised Standard Version Bible, copyright © 1989 Division of Christian Education of the National Council of the Churches of Christ in the United States of America. Used by permission. All rights reserved. The excerpt from "This Be the Verse" comes from *Collected Poems* by Philip Larkin. Copyright © 1988, 2003 by the Estate of Philip Larkin. Reprinted by permission of Farrar, Straus and Giroux, LLC, and Faber and Faber Ltd.

When I am doing philosophy well, or reading or listening to a very good philosopher, the experience is of discovering new, surprising, wonderful, and sometimes baffling depths and complications to existence, our lives, and our beliefs. Hardly a claim does not give way under its own pressure, calling for further thought and work. It can be exhausting, and it can be exhilarating. I am grateful to colleagues, friends, students, and some very fine referees for helping me in this work, encouraging me in it, and enjoying doing it with me.

Lydia Moland read and insightfully commented on all of the articles that led to this book. She also read a full draft of the manuscript and gave me a great number of helpful, subtle suggestions. Nancy Kelley was my advocate and mentor during seven years at Villanova University. It was a privilege, those same years, to be at the same institution as my father. His generosity to me has been boundless, his zeal for scholarly work that makes a difference an example since my youth.

My work also benefited from a brief stay at the Hastings Center as a visiting scholar in 2010. Daniel Callahan was my gracious host, and a proponent of the basic argument of this book. In 2011, colleagues at Villanova University, including Mark Doorley, Brett Wilmott, and Kathryn Getek, gave me helpful comments on an earlier version of chapter 1, and faculty in the Department of Philosophy at Boston College helped with some thoughtful questions in 2012. Adriaan Peperzak helped me to understand Kant better, for purposes of chapter 2; Colin Heydt helped me to understand better the language of rights, for purposes of chapters 2 and 5; and chapters 1, 3, 4, and 5 all benefited from presentation at meetings of the North American Society for Social Philosophy, where James Boettcher and Robert Murray were always cheerful conversation partners. Daniel Dahlstrom and William Desmond pushed me to synthesize my thinking into a book; some kind words about my work from Christopher Kaczor also helped in this regard. Honors students in a 2010 seminar at Villanova took joy in thinking about the matters covered in this book and convinced me that they were worth thinking through further. Fine colleagues at King's College—Joseph Evan, Gregory Bassham, and Regan Reitsma deserve special thanks—helped me to do just that.

After I had finished a full draft of this book, but while I was still struggling with the account of "what are parents for" in chapter 1, my mother died of amyotrophic lateral sclerosis, better known by its acronym, A.L.S. She had read and appreciated the article from which this chapter is drawn. Even in its improved form, however, it seems to me to provide but mute testimony of what she was to me and my sister.

Margaret has been my partner through thick and thin. I do not reflect in this book on what parents owe one another as, together, the parents of children. But I know that I owe her the dedication of this book, in deep gratitude and in recognition of all that she does to sustain and nourish our relationship well beyond any call of duty.

Introduction

It is perhaps only appropriate that a book on bringing children into being should have had a long gestation. This book was born of an uneasiness of mine, some years ago, with the literature on prenatal genetic enhancement and "engineering." To invoke an all-too-often discussed case, suppose that, given the richness of deaf culture as you and your partner have lived it, you wish to have a deaf child.[1] From your perspective, deafness counts as an enhancement: roughly, a characteristic that, duly cultivated, affords a person a richer life than otherwise might be expected. But is selecting for or in some sense "engineering" a deaf child morally permissible? In the literature on prenatal genetic enhancement, this question is typically answered by considering whether selecting for the desired characteristic would respect or violate the rights of the child-to-be.[2] In other words, what we find in this literature, which I discuss in my second-to-last chapter, is a generally unexamined presupposition that, so long as children's rights are respected (in particular children's so-called anticipatory autonomy rights), would-be parents may proceed as they wish. Yet surely, I felt, there must be more to say. One of the basic intuitions that gave rise to this book, then, is that respecting children's rights, or at least the oft-invoked right to an open future, is not "good enough." For the so-called good enough parent, to use the popular phrase, does much more.[3]

Another intuition that gave rise to this book is that we do better, in thinking about what parents owe children, to focus our attention first and foremost on parental obligations and not on children's rights, important though these are. We do better because, in the words of Onora O'Neill, whose work helped me move beyond intuitions, "when we take rights as fundamental in looking at ethical issues in children's lives we . . . get an indirect, partial and blurred picture."[4] More precisely, what we miss when we give pride of place in our thinking to children's rights is that parents and other adults may have so-called imperfect obligations to children that do not correspond to any rights on the part of children, or at most correspond to what earlier moralists called imperfect rights, a category that has fallen out of use.[5] O'Neill gives a helpful example:

> Although children cannot plausibly be said to have a *right* to the cheerful dailiness of family life, to some fun and attention, to some affection and understanding, most people would think that parents have a *responsibility*, an *obligation*, to provide a home and atmosphere which provides some (culturally specific) version of all these for their children, and that parents who do not do so fail in some of their basic obligations to their children.[6]

A parent who did so fail would accordingly fail to be, to use the popular phrase again, a good enough parent, and this despite the fact that the parent may have violated or neglected none of his or her child's rights (or at least "perfect" rights) and may in fact even be scrupulous about respecting these rights.

What I have called these intuitions of mine raise, however, a number of questions. To begin with, just what is the content of parental obligations, and how is this content determined? Further, how are parental obligations acquired—that is, what are the "grounds" of parental obligations—and who counts as a parent, which is to say who has parental obligations, in cases when a child is born through gamete donation or surrogacy (or, for that matter, cloning)? This book is the product of my working my way back from my intuitions and through the questions that they raise, which explains why the discussion of prenatal genetic enhancement comes not at the beginning of the book, but near its end.

The book's subtitle comes, as some readers might have recognized, from Mary Shelley's *Frankenstein*. Egregiously, it was not until some nine months *after* the animation of the creature that the good Dr. Frankenstein "[f]or the first time . . . felt what the duties of a creator towards his creature were."[7] To be clear, and lest there be any misunderstanding, I do not criticize the use of reproductive technologies as playing God (which, Shelley makes clear, Victor Frankenstein failed miserably at doing).[8] In other words, my drawing from Shelley's novel should not be understood as casting general suspicion on new ways of making babies. What I do share with Shelley, however, is an interest in the duties of parents as creators, or as I often put it "qua procreators." That is, I am interested in what parental obligations procreators incur by bringing children into being.

I do not speak, in this book, to the question of whether the parents who do the work of raising a child—parents who may be different from those who brought the child into being (the former may be termed social, the latter biological)—have parental obligations beyond those incurred by procreators. It could be that parents incur further obligations to a child by virtue of the relationship that they develop, and not only by virtue of having brought him or her into being.[9] As I do not speak to this question, I make no claim to be giving a full account of parental obligations, for perhaps there is more to say. What I claim to give is an account of the obligations that parents incur qua procreators. This account bears on the ethics of adoption, child support, gamete donation, surrogacy, and prenatal genetic enhancement—controversial topics, one and all, and all of which I go on to discuss in that order. (As I explain shortly, I do not, however, discuss the question of whether parents incur obligations to a child before his or her birth—a question that would bear, of course, on the ethics of abortion. My concern in this book is born children, not the unborn, and so I leave the ethics of abortion aside to the extent possible.)

The book consists of six chapters, though the last is less ambitious than the others and concerns a question that extends beyond the book's scope (namely, the question of public responsibility for children). In chapter 1, "What Are Parents For? A Thought Experiment," I pose a thought experiment. It has traditionally been held in cultures descended from the several Abrahamic religions that, while giving up a child can be morally permissible and may even be obligatory when the parents are for some reason incapable of raising him or her, giving up a child cannot be justified when there are not such extraordinary circumstances. In other words, giving up a child is permissible only when there are very good and pressing reasons.[10] But why? I pursue this question by asking why it would be wrong, if indeed it would be, for a couple to seek to have a child *with the idea in advance* of giving him or her up simply *at will*, which is to say without some good justification other than that they wanted to do so. (To put the same question in more current terms: why would it be wrong—if indeed it would be wrong—for a couple to plan to have to make an adoption or birth plan?) The question is admittedly strange, and it is difficult to imagine parents carrying through such a plan—unless, of course, we want to describe what surrogates do in these terms. In this chapter, however, I put surrogacy aside in order to press my question as a means of drawing out an account of "what are parents for," or in other words what obligations becoming a parent brings. (My focus, to reiterate, is on parents qua procreators.)

Chapter 1 comes to focus on the special nature and value of the relationship between procreators and children. The chapter closes, however, with a question: even acknowledging this special relationship, what reason is there to think that there is a prima facie, all-things-considered obligation for procreators to *develop* it? Two further questions arise in this context: that of the content of parental obligations and that of the "grounds," which is to say how parental obligations are acquired. There are two main positions in the literature on the question of the grounds. One, called the causal account of parental obligations, holds that one acquires parental obligations by having voluntarily acted in such a way that had the reasonably foreseeable consequence of bringing a child into being in the normal course of events. But this position is by no means uncontroversial. The main opposing position, called the voluntarist account, holds that one acquires parental obligations only by voluntarily assuming such obligations, whether explicitly or by so-called tacit acceptance. It might seem that the causal account has the support, for what it is worth, of conventional wisdom. For example, strict child support laws, now the rule in the United States, seem to presuppose it. Other practices like gamete donation and surrogacy, however, point in favor of the voluntarist account, as might the availability of abortion. For all these reasons and others as well, the voluntarist account has lately won strong support from philosophers. Defending the causal account, then, is no little undertaking.

My defense begins in chapter 2, "The Costs of Procreation." Here I defend and elaborate the causal account by considering, and countering, an argument that causal responsibility for the existence of a child brings with it the moral responsibility only to see to it that a child has what he or she needs in order to be protected from harm and enabled to live a minimally decent life. My own reckoning of what I call the costs of procreation is quite different and rather higher. I draw in this chapter from Seana Valentine Shiffrin's "equivocal view" of procreation—namely, that being brought into being is a mixed benefit, compromised by significant and inevitable burdens—in order to make the case that so-called procreative costs include the prima facie obligation to develop a loving parent-child relationship.

At this point, a reader might object, What about abortion? Is it not relevant that, when abortion is legal and available, a woman has a choice that a man does not, namely, whether to carry the pregnancy to term? To repeat from earlier in this introduction, my concern in this book is born children, not the unborn. I do not articulate a position, then, on the ethics of abortion as such or on the moral standing of the fetus. But the topic of abortion cannot be avoided altogether, because at least one well-known argument for the permissibility of abortion, namely, Judith Jarvis Thomson's famous "A Defense of Abortion," appears to undercut the causal account of parental obligations that chapter 2 elaborates and defends. And so chapter 3, "Abortion and the Grounds of Parental Obligations," is principally concerned with rebutting an argument from precedent that, if a woman does not acquire parental obligations to an unborn child just by having voluntarily acted in such a way that had the reasonably foreseeable consequence of bringing him or her into being, neither does a man acquire parental obligations to a child once he or she is born just by having voluntarily acted in the same way. (Thomson grants, for the sake of argument, that a fetus has the full moral standing of a person; hence my referring to it as an unborn child.) This chapter is, I think, the most "technical" and demanding in the book, but it concerns questions that can more or less be predicted to arise in this context and that defy quick and easy understanding. To repeat one last time, I do not articulate here a position on the ethics of abortion.[11] Instead, I am concerned with defending the viability of the causal account of parental obligations.

The following chapter takes up the puzzling question of just who has parental obligations in cases where gamete donation or surrogacy has been used to bring a child into being. To put the question differently, is gamete donation or surrogacy rightly considered cost free? More briefly, I ask here, in the terms of the chapter's title, "Whose Child?" Critics of the causal account claim that it is useless for the purpose of assigning parental responsibility when gamete donation or surrogacy has been used. For the causal account "fingers too many people," or in other words "spreads parental responsibility too widely."[12] Accordingly, proponents of the voluntarist account point to these practices as prime exhibits of the folly of the causal account and as evidence for the voluntarist account: to quote one such proponent, "think of sperm donors!"[13] In this chapter, I counter that the causal account is not quite so hopeless as its critics claim, and claim instead that it provides us a principled, reasonable way to come to terms with both gamete donation and surrogacy. Further, I subject both these practices to critical scrutiny in the light of my arguments from chapters 1 and 2.

With chapter 5, "Good Enough Parenting?" the focus turns to the ethics of prenatal genetic enhancement. As I have already noted, the literature on prenatal genetic enhancement is typically focused on the importance of preserving children's anticipatory autonomy rights, formulated in brief as the right to an open future. My chapter critically examines arguments for this right, which was first developed in reaction to the United States Supreme Court's 1972 *Yoder* decision on the education of children. I do not reject the child's right to an open future, but draw attention to the limits of its proponents' understanding of children's interests. Accordingly, what I do reject is the position that respecting this right is "good enough"—that, so long as the child's right to an open future is respected, would-be parents may do as they wish. To be clear, I do not oppose all prenatal genetic enhancements, or for that matter propose that any or all should be outlawed. But I think that there are good reasons to be wary. Like some other authors, my concern with technologies that promise parental choice of children's genetic characteristics is not principally that they might violate children's rights—though perhaps some could well— but that they might lead a parent to assess children as products of his or her will and design and so cut against the normative unconditionality of the parent-child relationship. In other words, choice of a child's genetic characteristics could render a parent's love all too conditional: namely, on the child's satisfying parental expectations. To close the chapter, I consider objections to this argument and, in so doing, develop it further.

The book's sixth and final chapter takes us, as its title indicates, back from the futuristic prospect of prenatal genetic enhancement to a more contemporary and mundane question. As the sociologist Viviana Zelizer has observed, the twentieth century saw a "profound cultural transformation in children's economic and sentimental value": in brief, "the priceless child displaced the useful child."[14] The so-called sacralization of children's lives was surely for the better—who would argue that children *ought* to be viewed as economic assets, or that child labor is in itself a good thing?—but the transformation did not come without costs, especially for poorer families. Not only do today's children cost parents much and give back little economically;[15] what's more, the great value that we place on children of our *own* has gone hand-in-hand with what Zelizer terms a "collective indifference to other people's children."[16] Children have become, in brief, a private luxury,[17] reflected in the fact that "child support awards in America are often just high enough to enable a single mother to avoid welfare, but not high enough to ensure that her children obtain an adequate standard of living."[18] To close this book, I consider what ought to be the policy implications of the great value that we place in our society on our *own* children. My aim is to bring into focus a question that, admittedly, extends beyond the scope of this book: the question of public responsibility for children (in terms of the chapter's title, who should pay for the priceless child).

As I have already noted, the topics considered in this book—the ethics of adoption, child support, gamete donation, surrogacy, and prenatal genetic enhancement—are all controversial. They are also, I think, philosophically rich and challenging, as well as now and again quite troubling. My hope is that readers will share my appreciation of these topics, without losing sight of the human consequences of how we come to answer the philosophical questions that they raise. I also hope that readers will be inspired to pursue some of these questions further. The many authors whom I quote and cite—sometimes to criticize, sometimes to advance my own thinking—have produced a variegated and lively body of literature, full of insights and questions beyond those taken up here. There are two reasons to recommend the literature on procreative ethics and parental obligations. The first is that the rigorous, self-critical thinking that this literature exhibits and demands may lay the foundation for sounder practices in the matters it addresses. The second, I think, is that the discipline of rigorous, self-critical thinking about matters of importance is valuable itself.

1 What Are Parents For?
A Thought Experiment

As Milton's Adam observes in a fit of pique after his fall from grace, one of the things that parents do for children—analogizing God as father and mother both—is to presume to bring them into being. (When I refer to parents in the following, I normally have in mind parents qua pro-creators, as the context should make clear.) Neither informed consent, nor even mere assent is, of course, possible on the part of children-to-be. Moreover, once we are here, whenever that strange and remarkable event occurs in our development, there is no not having been here, and there is also no easy means of exit should we not be happy with the course that our lives are taking. In Adam's words (in verse that reappears, signifi-cantly, as the epigraph to Shelley's *Frankenstein*):

> Did I request thee, Maker, from my clay
> To mould me Man? Did I solicit thee
> From darkness to promote me . . .?[1]

The lament is ancient. Nietzsche refers to the "ancient story" of Midas's capture of Silenus—and Silenus's cackle that "'[w]hat is best for [human beings] is beyond [our] reach forever: not to be born, not to *be*, to be *nothing*.'"[2] Job wishes that his creation could be undone in language that inverts the creation story in Genesis 1:

> Let the day perish in which I
> was born.
> and the night that said,
> "A man-child is conceived."
> Let that day be darkness!
> May God above not seek it,
> or light shine on it.
> Let gloom and deep darkness
> claim it.[3]

Philip Larkin's vision in his oft-quoted poem "This Be the Verse" is funnier but perhaps even darker. I pass over the infamous first line (which as a rule is all that is ever quoted) for the final stanza:

> Man hands on misery to man.
> It deepens like a coastal shelf.
> Get out as early as you can.
> And don't have any kids yourself.[4]

This last bit of advice is presumably for "the good of the child"; the poet or, in any event, the poem appears to deem all human life wrongful life.[5] It is, obviously, an extreme judgment, and most bioethicists do not go nearly so far.[6] Then there are the paradoxes that cluster under the bristling name of the non-identity problem. These appear to dissolve the worry that parents can *harm* a child in bringing him or her into being, and so absolve would-be parents of any culpability for a child's existence in all instances but when it can be predicted that the child's life would be so terrible that it would not even be worth living.[7] The non-identity problem takes its name from the supposition that "in different outcomes"—for example, when parents conceive a child now though this child will have a disability (outcome 1) rather than delaying several months, in order for the problem in question to pass, and having a child without this disability (outcome 2)—"different people would exist."[8] In these different outcomes, to restate the point in different terms, the people who stand to come into being would not be identical with one another. Accordingly, it is not the case that the child with the disability might have been brought into being without this disability if only her parents had delayed trying to conceive; instead, if her parents had delayed, this child would never have existed at all. The only way for her to come into being was to come into being with her disability; and so (here is the kicker) it appears not to make any sense to say that her parents *harmed* her, which is to say acted against her interests, though they knew that she would come into being disabled. If we want to say that the parents committed some crime, it appears to be a crime without a victim. For the only alternative for the child, to speak nonsense for a moment, would be never to have come into being—which is nonsense since nonexistence is obviously no alternative *for her*.[9] Yes, nonexistence might be *preferable* for her if we could predict that she would not have a "life worth living"—if the "bads" of that life would overwhelm any goods in it, or her existence were so terrible that it constituted an evil to her; but no, existence would not be *worse* for her than never having existed—she would not, strictly speaking, have been *harmed* in being summoned from darkness to light, to recall the imagery deployed by Adam and Job.

In bioethics, the non-identity problem is often deployed against those who, in the interests of children, would put limits on would-be parents' reproductive liberty. In other words, it appears, not as a problem to be solved or circumvented, but as an *argument* used to dismiss objections to reproductive decisions made before a child is conceived or very early in its development. For example, according to John Harris, "[t]here is no complaint the 'victim' of gender selection [or surrogacy, or artificial insemination by donor, or cloning] can make because for her there was no alternative but never to have existed." In fact, he goes on,

> the same is true for any significant genetic manipulation that might be made to an embryo or indeed to the gametes prior to conception, if this ever becomes possible. So complaints that parents who would use gender selection are attempting to shape or mold their children [and thereby potentially harming them] are simply incoherent. [The parents] may of course be choosing what sorts of children will come into existence, but none of those children have any legitimate or even coherent complaint, for they could not have had an alternative life free of such externally imposed choices.[10]

Yet not all objections to reproductive decisions need turn on the interests of the children so produced; the non-identity problem, retooled as an argument,[11] does appear to undercut this kind of objection, but only this kind. It is a basic thesis of this book that parents, qua procreators, have obligations regarding future children that constrain the liberty of would-be parents to do as they wish. Moreover, these obligations go beyond respecting the oft-invoked child's right to an open future (discussed in chapter 5). If it is objected that a person cannot have the obligations of a parent until a child, in fact, exists, the reply should be that, while *yes* a person would not have obligations to the child until she exists, a person is obligated *not* to create a child unless that person has a reasonable belief that he or she will be capable of carrying out the relevant obligations and is committed in advance to doing so. Analogously, a person does not have the obligation to repay a debt until he or she in fact borrows money. But that person would be wrong to borrow the money without a reasonable belief that he or she could repay the debt and without being committed in advance to the repayment.[12] The upshot is that, if we have reason to think that a reproductive decision would lead to the violation of parental obligations, then we can object to this decision without having to engage the paradoxes of the non-identity problem.[13] Whether the parents who bring a child into being thereby incur the obligation to do any of the work of parenting *themselves* is a further question that this chapter goes on to investigate.

One way to elaborate my thesis is to think about adoption, and so this chapter proposes to do so. As Jonathan Glover has observed, the model of adoption is potentially misleading for thinking about reproductive decisions.[14] For the child who is available for adoption already exists and so decisions concerning this child—for example, with what parents to place him or her—can harm his or her interests; not so the child who cannot come into being but in *this* particular condition with *these* particular parents. I want, however, to come at adoption from a different angle. It has traditionally been held, at least in cultures shaped by the several Abrahamic religions, that what can be permitted and may be the better course *in extremis*—namely, giving up a child—cannot be justified in ordinary circumstances, which is to say when there are not very good and pressing reasons, even if one could be confident that another individual or for that matter institution could do the job of raising one's child just as well or even better.[15] In other words, so-called abandonment—richly studied by the historian John Boswell in his book *The Kindness of Strangers*—is justifiable in some circumstances, but not all circumstances, again even if others could do the job just as well or even better.[16] But why? I put the question this way: why would it be wrong—if indeed it would be wrong—for a couple to seek to conceive a child *with the idea*, in advance, of giving him or her up simply *at will*, which is to say without some reason other than that they wanted to do so? (In more current terms: why would it be wrong—if indeed it would be wrong—for a couple to plan to have to make an adoption or birth plan?) Trying to answer this question requires us to think about, not just what parents do for children, like presume to bring them into being, but what obligations becoming a parent brings: in the colloquial terms of this chapter's title, "what are parents for." Once we have this account, which I think would be valuable in and of itself for our appreciation of the role of parent, we can go on to consider in chapters to come whether, or under what circumstances, new ways of becoming a parent now and in the future—through gamete donation, surrogacy, and prenatal genetic enhancement—are likely to be compatible with the obligations of parents, qua procreators, to children. But first, in this chapter and the next, there is no little groundwork to be done. To prepare the reader, my argument in this chapter takes more than one twist and turn, and it is not until chapter 2 that the argument comes to a close.

§1. THE TRADITION AND TWO ANSWERS

Alan Donagan articulates what he calls the "precept of parental responsibility" in the Hebrew-Christian tradition as follows: "It is impermissible for human beings voluntarily to become parents of a child, and yet to refuse to rear it to a stage of development at which it can independently take part in social life."[17] He further remarks that "[f]or a child whose natural parents cannot assume this authority, for any reason from death to temperamental unfitness, other arrangements must be made, for example, adoption; but they are considered to be intrinsically inferior."[18] Parental obligations or duties are then what are termed *prima facie*, which is to say obligations or duties that obtain not absolutely, but on the condition that there are not overriding considerations.[19] In other words, according at least to the Hebrew-Christian tradition, procreators are prima facie obligated to parent the children whom they bring into being and so to carry out the duties of parenthood, whatever they may be (which at this point I do not presume to say). Remarkably, Jewish, Islamic, and the common law do not even have the category of adoption and instead only foster care. By contrast, "Modern American law (like the Code of Hammurabi, Roman law, and the Napoleonic code) has full legal adoption."[20] The 1851 Massachusetts Act to Provide for the Adoption of Children, which became the model statute across the United States, declared the adopted child "the same to all intents and purposes as if such child had been born in lawful wedlock of such parents or parent by adoption," while terminating the so-called natural parents' "legal rights . . . as respects such child" and freeing him or her "from all legal obligations of maintenance and obedience, as respects such natural parent or parents."[21] The growing practice of open adoption since the 1980s is, of course, introducing significant changes to this model as well as challenges to the adoptive family; but the background for these changes and challenges is adoption understood more or less as the Massachusetts act conceived it.[22]

Given the great changes in matters familial and sexual over the last fifty-plus years, it might come as a surprise that the traditional precept that Donagan articulates appears more or less to reflect common morality today, at least within cultures descended from the Abrahamic religions. Though it is legally permitted, giving up a child for adoption when one is competent to care for the child and there is nothing untoward in one's life circumstances is seen as morally suspect.[23] Donagan's claim that other arrangements like adoption are "intrinsically inferior" to rearing by birth parents has not fared as well, though it has perhaps fared better than it should. Recent empirical research supports the view that, as Elizabeth Bartholet puts it, adoption "should be recognized as a positive form of family, not ranked as a poor imitation of the real thing on some parenting hierarchy."[24] After all, a child's birth parents may prove terrible, and it can be a mercy to be given into the care of others, even the care of strangers. In any event, the current consensus appears to be that giving up a child for adoption may be commendable—indeed, it can be seen as "the last in a series of actions meant to provide care for the child"[25]—but must also be undertaken with great seriousness.[26]

At least one contemporary practice—namely, surrogacy—may well tell a different story,[27] but I want to put it aside for now in order to focus instead on my question of why it would be wrong, if indeed it would be, for a *couple* to seek to conceive a child with the idea of giving him or her up simply at will, which is the case neither in so-called traditional surrogacy (where the mother contributes both genes and gestation) nor in gestational surrogacy (where the mother contributes "only" gestation).

Admittedly, the question is somewhat strange, perhaps even disturbing: for many birth parents, the decision to give up a child is traumatic, even tragic in some sense. As Paul Lauritzen has observed in a thoughtful and well-documented discussion, "many children surrendered for adoption are not in fact unwanted by their biological parents, but are relinquished anyway because there is no alternative" in the face of unrelenting poverty,[28] which was likewise often the case when children were "abandoned" in Antiquity and the Middle Ages.[29] It should also be acknowledged that giving up a child has proven quite difficult for some surrogates, as several highly publicized court cases might be called on to attest.[30] All the same, I propose that thinking about the question of why it would be wrong, etc., can prove instructive. For it calls on us to think more deeply than we typically do about both the grounds and content of procreators' obligations to children. (Note that, in this chapter, I do not distinguish among procreators, birth parents, and biological or genetic parents. Once we turn from the case of a couple conceiving a child to consider procreation through gamete donation and surrogacy, these terms will need to be pried apart.)

One of the few authors who has spoken to my question, though briefly, is Leon Kass. According to him:

> We practice adoption because there are abandoned children who need good homes. We do not, and would not, encourage people deliberately to generate children for others to adopt, partly because we wish to avoid baby markets, partly because we think it unfair to deliberately deprive the child of his natural ties.[31]

So here are two possible answers to why it would be wrong for a couple to seek to conceive a child with the idea of giving him or her up: first, interpreting somewhat, it would reduce the child to a thing, or in Kantian language a mere means to some purpose (in a word, sale);[32] and, second, it would deprive the child of "his natural ties," or what Kass also calls a knowledge of his "roots." Such knowledge, Kass claims, is of "profound importance . . . for self-identity." "Clarity about your origins," he writes, "is crucial for self-identity, itself important for self-respect."[33]

To speak to the first answer: would a child who had been conceived with the idea of giving him or her up, whether for money as in some surrogacy arrangements or as a gift in adoption, necessarily be treated merely as a means and not also as an end in him or herself (that is, someone whose own good deserves respect)? This conclusion, which is often drawn in discussions of traditional surrogacy, might seem inevitable. In the rather strong words of one author, such surrogate mother arrangements, "of necessity, treat the creation of a person as the means to the gratification of the interests of others, rather than respect the child as an end in himself." The surrogate mother, "[b]y the very nature of the transaction," cannot "make a pretense to valuing the child in and for himself, since she would not otherwise be creating the child but for the monetary and other . . . considerations [that] she receives under the surrogate mother contract."[34]

Once we think some, however, about the meaning of the Kantian imperative to treat persons "always at the same time as an end and never merely as a means,"[35] then the judgment that the child is necessarily treated merely as a means appears less certain. On one common interpretation, "We use others as *mere means* if what we do reflects some maxim [that is, policy] *to which they could not in principle consent.*"[36] Paradigmatic examples include deception, coercion, and violence. In deceiving someone, one involves another in a project to which he or she cannot in principle consent, since it must be concealed; in coercing someone, one makes someone do something to which he or she cannot in principle consent, since he or she has no real choice; and in doing violence to someone, one attacks and damages or destroys another's very capacity to give consent. Now, it is not at all obvious that a child conceived with the idea of giving him or her up *could not in principle* consent—though only after the fact, of course—to the maxim on which his or her mother is acting. It is true that we cannot presume his or her consent to such a way of coming into being, which might well make for a difficult life; but this is a different kind of objection (it does not challenge the permissibility of the action on Kantian grounds), which what's more appears vulnerable to the non-identity problem. Imagine John Harris asking: just how bad a life would it likely be? And then telling the child: you have no legitimate or even coherent complaint. Seeking to conceive a child with the idea of giving him or her up does not, then, appear wrong on the Kantian ground that it treats the child merely as a means.

Perhaps, though, a surrogate treats the child merely as a means in some less technical, non-Kantian sense: after all, whether we want to say that she is paid for the child or paid for carrying and then birthing him or her, the surrogate does have the child for some purpose to which the child is subordinate. In brief, the child is "just used" by the surrogate. Commercial surrogacy uneasily mixes what Virginia Held calls "the paradigm of economic man," who organizes life in contractual terms, with "the paradigm of mother and child," bound by affection.[37] It is not obvious, however, that having a child for some purpose to which the child is subordinate is necessarily wrong. Imagine a woman or man who agrees to have a child with his or her partner in order, principally or even exclusively, to make that child-loving partner happy. Though the child is "just used" in this regard, doing so does not appear wrong, and the child is in fact valued as an end by at least one party to this decision, namely, the partner who desperately wants him or her. (In more technical terms, the child-loving partner sees the child as a nonderivative source of reasons: the reason to have a child is not derived from consideration of other reasons, as it is for the other partner.[38]) Likewise, in surrogacy arrangements, at least one party values the child as an end, namely, the parents or parent who takes this child as his or her own. So in sum: the first possible answer to why it would be wrong to seek to conceive a child with the idea of giving him or her up does not appear sufficient. For the child so conceived is not necessarily treated merely as a means in a morally objectionable way. (There is of course much more to say about surrogacy; I focus on *commercial* surrogacy at some length in chapter 4.)

To speak to the second answer: Kass does not explain why knowledge of roots, or clarity about origins, is so important for self-identity, but it seems right to say that such knowledge does matter deeply to some people, though not to all.[39] In any event, as another author has noted in analyzing the language both of professionals and of "*some* adopted children," the problem here is certainly not the problem of personal identity discussed by philosophers like Locke and Hume.[40] Instead, the literature tends to refer to psychologist Erik Erikson's conception of identity as "*confidence* in one's inner continuity amid change."[41] On this account, to have an identity means to be secure in who one is, or in other words, again speaking somewhat colloquially, to have a strong sense of self.[42] Yet this kind of identity, some claim, is precisely what adopted persons lack. In the words of a leader of what has come to be called the search movement:

> Adopted children have little continuity in their lives; for the most part, they have been cut off from, or have little knowledge of, the past. Their identities are fragile—whether they are adopted as newborns or later—and have been shaped by the trauma of separation from the birth mother, as well as by feelings of abandonment and the lack of a coherent life narrative.[43]

We need to be wary, however, of agreeing too quickly with such claims. It is striking that advocates of the so-called new psychology of the adopted, like the activist quoted, show little awareness of what another author has termed "the cultural contexts in which [experiences of adoption] are embedded," but freely make claims about adopted persons' universal needs.[44] If some adopted persons disagree about these needs, they are characterized as repressed.[45] The story of "the search," motivated by the sense that "something is missing," has become a common tale in recent years, part of the pathologizing of adoption that has gone hand in hand with the return of an obsession with genetics.[46] Though Kass would be horrified to hear it, his equation of "natural ties" with biological ties appears to belong to this trend. By contrast, as two critics of Kass's argument have observed, "natural connection"—connection that deepens as the child grows up—"might also be created through needs-fulfillment."[47] In other words, rearing too might create deeply rooted relationships and so give a child a deeply rooted sense of self.

There are, of course, multiple reasons why adopted persons search for their birth parents, including to gain information about genetic health history and to come to terms with "concerns about why they were 'given away' or 'given up.'"[48] *Pace* the "new psychology of the adopted," however, knowledge of biological ties does not appear in all cases essential for a person to have a strong sense of self, though some adopted persons do at times feel a strong need for this knowledge (for example, before beginning a family themselves); and the need should not be dismissed as "merely" a cultural artifact—as if, were the need "merely" cultural in origin, it would thereby be less real. Whether it would be wrong deliberately to bring into being a child who would be deprived of this knowledge, or would need to search it out, is certainly debatable.[49] One way or the other, though, this objection does not seem to go quite to the heart of the matter.

§2. THE GIVEN RELATIONSHIP

It might appear that we have not gotten very far toward answering my question (why would it be wrong for a couple to seek to conceive a child with the idea of giving him or her up), but I want to consider further the reasons why adopted persons search for their birth parents. I listed two motivations: to gain information about genetic health history, and to come to terms with "concerns about why they were 'given away' or 'given up.'" Now, persons whose adoptions were open instead of closed, as most adoptions used to be, do not typically have these motivations: the genetic information is already available, and they often know why their birth parents chose adoption.[50] Yet it is remarkable that many of these persons search for their birth parents nonetheless. (Some, of course, know and have relationships with them already.) According to several researchers, "As more information is shared with children, it . . . does not negate curiosity about their birthparents. . . . During adolescence, this curiosity can lead to strong intentions to search and searching behavior."[51] Why?

It ought to be acknowledged that the answer might simply be adolescent angst. In other words, perhaps the adolescent who searches for his or her birth parents has simply latched onto the fact that is most mysterious about him or herself, comparable to an adolescent who becomes fascinated with, say, a parent's abandoned culture or religion.[52] But the reasons appear to go deeper, as suggested by the fact that the desire to discover one's birth parents is attested in cultures unacquainted with our teenage wastelands or the figure of the adolescent.[53]

Onora O'Neill has suggested another answer: "It is evident," she writes, "that given relationships matter deeply to people."[54] By "given," understand relationships that cannot be undone, or that have an ineluctable permanence. Paradigmatic examples include the non-adoptive parent-child relationship and that between siblings: the biological ties cannot be broken, though of course the relationships may be emotionally broken or severed in other ways. The contrast is with chosen relationships, the paradigmatic examples of which include friendship and modern-day marriage. In given relationships, the parties need to work on the relationship to make it happy, but it is there, at least in a sense, whether they work on it or not. In chosen relationships, the parties typically need to work to make the relationship happy if it is to be there at all, which is to say if it is not to dissolve altogether.[55] To put the point in brief, persons can be former friends, but not former siblings. As evidence of the profound importance of given relationships to people, O'Neill observes that

> adopted persons, even when they have had happy childhoods and love their adoptive parents, often want to make contact with their birth parents. Often they speak of the longing to know their birth parents as becoming stronger over the years, and as particularly strong when they have children of their own. . . . They may also want to know of and to know any (half) brothers and sisters, or any other genetic relatives. Although one often hears of adopted parents who explain to their children that they were *chosen*, this fact clearly does not always expunge the sense of loss, the sense that *from the child's point of view*, it would have been better *not* to have been chosen, but given.[56]

Why given relationships matter so much to people is another question. To begin with, these relationships provide the *setting* for our lives: they give us the terms through which we may place ourselves—for example, as the child of these parents, or as the sibling of these brothers or sisters—an echo of Kass's observation about the importance of knowledge of "roots."[57] Further, as Claudia Mills has observed, given or what she terms unchosen relationships form a bed for the development of relationships marked by unconditional love—more fully and precisely, love that attaches more to a person's being, to the sheer fact of the person's existence, than to his or her features or accomplishments and failures.[58] By way of example (for there is no denying that this love is rather mysterious), it is a remarkable fact that an expectant parent can love a child before he or she is even born, which is to say before the parent knows much at all about the child, including whether the child is a he or a she. This kind of love is based more on the child's *being* (yet more precisely, the child's being the parent's) than on any characteristics that he or she has or will develop. Barring confusion at the hospital over whose child is whose, or deception over paternity, the one "condition" of this kind of love is not a condition that could be disappointed and so in a sense is not a condition at all: it is the given relationship between the parent and child, that the child is the parent's and the parent is the child's.

Joseph Kupfer has insightfully suggested that the ground of the unconditional love of parents for children may be what he calls parents' *identification* with their children: the fact that a child's well-being and suffering "is experienced as constitutive of [a parent's] own well-being and suffering."[59] For the loving parent, the child is "another oneself," to use Aristotle's characterization of the friend, in a way deeper than even the friend is. Again to explain by way of example, whereas friends grieve with us, "parents don't just grieve with us; they also grieve for us," and so need consoling from *their* friends when their children suffer.[60] In the ideal, a parent loves a child in much the same way and on much the same grounds that the parent loves him or herself: not conditionally, but as part and parcel of his or her being. (We could also say, I think, by virtue of being.) Kupfer further claims, and here too I find him insightful, that the love of child for parent is, even in the ideal, not this same unconditional love. Instead, ideally, a child's love for his or her parent is grounded in the child's gratitude to the parent—gratitude for the fact that the parent has proved "a protecting, nurturing, unconditionally *loving* authority."[61] Of course, there should be no illusion that the ideal of parental love is always realized. To repeat, given or unchosen relationships form a bed for the development of relationships marked by unconditional love. In other words, they hold this potential, which may or may not be actualized. It should also be recognized that what we call unconditional love is in fact fragile and perhaps rarer than we might like to think. One philosopher has us imagine a child who proves rapist, serial killer, or torturer.[62] As the pain of a thankless, or worse, older child may break the human heart, when I speak of unconditional love in the following, I mean love that is unconditional to the extent that is humanly possible.

An important question to consider here is what role a child's being the parents' own—that is, the given relationship between parents and child—plays in the parents' coming to love the child by virtue of his or her being (otherwise put, as they love themselves). In other words, how does the biological tie lead to or at least support parents' identification with their child? A plausible answer, I think, is that parents come to identify with a child because they see him or her (indeed, for the mother especially, experience him or her) as an extension of themselves: in poetic terms, bone of our bone, flesh of our flesh. The child is naturally seen as "another oneself" because he or she bears and shows forth the parents' own life, individually and as one flesh themselves.

Why it is important that children *enjoy* given relationships—more precisely, that children have relationships as they grow up that they can count on *as* given, whether these relationships have any biological component or not—is suggested already by the preceding reflections. To quote O'Neill again, "knowledge that the parent will persist"—will stick with or stand by the parent-child relationship—"is of great importance to a child's . . . sense of security and belonging."[63] Moreover, the normative unconditionality of the parent-child relationship (note that this unconditionality holds for the parent, not the child) gives a child a sense that he or she is of great value, which is to say so valuable that the parent will not give up on him or her for any but the most trying causes.[64] (The child who proves serial killer or torturer makes it clear that, while unconditionality is the rule, the application of the rule has its limits.) It is noteworthy in this regard that a "sense of rejection . . . usually accompanies most parent-child separations" and that "the sense of rejection, of not being wanted or being a 'cast-off,' seems to undermine [some adopted] children's sense of self-esteem and self-worth,"[65] even when they have been lucky enough to find, or more precisely to be found by, parents who provide love and acceptance. It should immediately be added, however, that not giving up on the relationship does not exclude letting the child go, or making him or her leave, should the child's behavior make living with that child extremely difficult or practically impossible. What is distinctive to a relationship that can be counted on *as* given is that the *offer* of the relationship is always there. The parent in such a relationship is committed *in principle* to the relationship even when facts on the ground stand in its way.[66]

Note that I do *not* claim that *parental* love is essential to a child's flourishing. Studies indicate that some measure of affection, from someone, is necessary for a child to flourish in even the minimal sense of developing basic human capacities within a normal range;[67] and it makes sense to think that parents are the most reliable, though as we know by no means foolproof, sources of such affection. Happily, however, the love of a nurse or a nanny, or a sibling or a social worker or an extraordinary teacher, may prove enough for a child who has the great misfortune either of losing her parents, or of having parents who fail to love her. Yet, even if the child finds the love that she needs elsewhere, not having parents or having parents who fail to love her is still a great misfortune: there is nothing "happy" about it. For she would nonetheless be deprived of the special goods of a healthy parent-child relationship, goods that would contribute greatly to her welfare or well-being, considerations of flourishing and its proper description apart.

The notion of special goods has been developed by Simon Keller in a discussion of filial duty. In Keller's terms, what makes special goods "special" in this context is that they are goods that a parent or a child "can receive from no one (or almost no one)" but one another. Special goods are distinguished from generic goods, "which could in principle be received from anyone."[68] Love is a good that is generic in this sense, but parental love is obviously a good that could not be had from just anyone. Moreover, there are reasons to think that a life would be significantly less rich—more strongly, even significantly impoverished—without the special good of parental love.[69] From the point of view of the child, the special goods of a healthy parent-child relationship include having a person who, having known you intimately since your birth or in any event early childhood, may know, understand, and sympathize with you in ways that others cannot, and indeed in some ways may even know you better than you know yourself; having someone not only who is committed to your well-being, but whose well-being is tightly bound up with yours; having someone who can be counted on to be there for you in a way that you cannot count on most others, not excluding friends and romantic partners and increasingly even spouses; and, in brief, having someone who loves you unconditionally, simply because you are you, that person's child.[70] Without these special goods and this kind of love, life would be a lonelier, more forbidding undertaking.[71]

I think that we can now return to my question (why would it be wrong, etc.) with a better chance of making headway. Here is a first go at an answer: while making an adoption plan *is* justifiable when, during a pregnancy, parents realize that they cannot provide for the child as they are obligated to do, for a couple to seek to conceive a child *with the idea* of giving him or her up simply at will appears to be wrong for two reasons: first, it exposes the child to the risk of potentially debilitating feelings of rejection; second, it treats as a thing of little value something that is potentially of tremendous value and importance to a child, namely, the given or unchosen relationship with his or her birth parents (that is, procreators). To reiterate, the value of such a relationship lies in the fact that it forms a bed for the development of a relationship marked by unconditional love—love that attaches to the child's being, the sheer fact of his or her existence. In other words, a relationship that is given or unchosen can serve as the basis for a relationship that can be counted on *as* given—a relationship offering a child great goods that can scarcely be had from anyone other than a parent.

§3. THE TRANSFER PRINCIPLE

This answer needs, however, some further consideration. To begin with, it bears repeating that adoptive parents, too, can certainly provide a child a relationship that can be counted on *as* given, and so it seems reasonable to think that adoptive parents can at least minimize the risk of a child's suffering debilitating feelings of rejection. Moreover, though the relationship does not have any biological component and so is not "given" in this sense—the child is not "bone of our bones, flesh of our flesh"—there is an important sense in which, typically, the relationship is nonetheless unchosen. (The terms 'given' and 'unchosen' here diverge.) Putting aside the use of genetic technologies, just as biological parents may choose to seek to have a child, but do not choose the particular child they welcome into the world, adoptive parents choose to seek to have a child, but in the end must simply live with, and discover and come to terms with, the child they welcome into their home. Yes, like biological parents, adoptive parents might know in advance some of a child's gross characteristics, but in fact, at least when the child in question is an infant or very young, they exercise little choice over the nature of the particular child whom they take as their own. Instead, surely the most significant fact about this child for expectant adoptive parents, no less than for expectant biological parents, is simply that he or she is to be *theirs*, in the profound sense of theirs to rear and raise. Adoptive parents may not be able to see their child as bone of their bones, flesh or their flesh, but they can nonetheless deeply identify with him or her, who after all goes forth into the world by virtue of their labor.

Along these same lines, it should be underscored that what we really value here is the unconditional love of parents for children. Just how a child came to be one's *own*, which is to say whether through procreation or adoption, appears not all that important (so long as, of course, the child did not become one's own illegally). What is important is that a love develop that is based more on the child's *being* than on any characteristics that he or she has or will come to have. Such a love, after all, could overcome even confusion at the hospital over whose child is whose, or deception over paternity.[72] In this regard, I think that Paul Lauritzen is right that, "while genetic connection may foster relational bonds, it is the bonds that are crucial, not the genetic ties." In other words, "it is the ongoing, caring relationship with a child that is the core of responsible parenthood."[73]

In the end, we need to come to terms with what Tim Bayne calls "*the transfer principle*, according to which it is permissible to alienate one's parental responsibilities (over neonates) to another individual (or institution) as long as one has good reason to think that [the individual or institution] will carry out those responsibilities adequately," without need for further justification, such as that one is mentally or financially incapable of meeting the responsibilities oneself.[74] At the bottom of the transfer principle is the supposition that what procreators owe a child is to see to it that he or she is cared for, not necessarily to care for the child themselves.[75]

I can think of two reasons to be wary of the transfer principle—though note that I do not say to reject it altogether (a point to which I return in chapter 4, in discussing gamete donation and surrogacy). The first reason is that, while procreators can extract from others the *promise* of commitment, they cannot extract the thing itself.[76] After all, part of the trauma of adoption is that whether unconditionally loving parents will be found is a matter of chance. Once the child is relinquished, even in open adoptions, how the child is raised is at least largely if not entirely out of the birth parents' hands. In a word, this objection is epistemic (that is, having to do with the limits of knowledge). What makes it vulnerable, however, is that it is built on a denial of what the transfer principle takes for granted: that one has "good reason" to think that one's child will be well cared for. Yes, birth parents can never know for sure, but if the adoption is arranged through a public agency, with diligent screening, a thorough home visit, and the supervision of competent social workers, it might be claimed that worry in this regard is unmotivated—worry more "in principle" than rooted in fact.[77]

This defense is strong, but I do not think we should be overly impressed. It is surely correct that a parent who with good reason does not believe him or herself capable of meeting parental obligations does right in surrendering her child to "an organized social scheme of child adoption with an assured historic record of general success."[78] In such a case, the interests of an existing child speak for taking the chance that his or her life, too, will count among the successes. But it does not follow that this "historic record of general success" would likewise justify the plan of a couple who seek to conceive a child with the idea of giving him or her up (the case, to recall, that got this discussion going). They take a chance that did not need to be taken—more precisely, that the interests of an existing child did not call for—which it is then difficult to see as justifiable. The transfer principle is quite blithe about the likelihood of coming to know that one has "good reason" to entrust others with the demanding, and sometimes draining, responsibilities of raising a child. It might be objected in turn that one cannot be certain about one's own future commitment to these responsibilities, but this objection seems specious: one can hold oneself accountable in ways that one cannot hold others.

The second reason to be wary of the transfer principle goes deeper. This is that, when all is said and done, the transfer principle does not take into account the value of the given, biological relationship. Again precision is needed: the transfer principle does not take into account the value that the given, biological relationship is accorded in societies like ours, with roughly our concept and institution of the family, where being bone of another's bones, flesh of another's flesh is a relationship of great significance. (By way of contrast, consider the relationship of simply having the same blood type as another person.) Now, it could well be asked whether the importance of this relationship is merely "socially constructed," and thus relative to this or that society, or universally valid, say a fact of human nature. Imagine, by way of counterexample, a world in which adoption is the norm. Would adopted children experience angst in such a world?[79] I think that the right answer to this question is: we have no idea, for it is not a world with which we are familiar. Not all societies, of course, have or have had the same concept and institution of the family, though all societies have some analogous institution.[80] I am not writing, however, for all times and places. Instead, my concern in this book is with the ethics of the family as we know it—"we" being, roughly, contemporaries who live in societies where the questions that this chapter has been pursuing make sense. In the world that we know, with our kinship structures, the importance of the biological relationship is a matter of course. It is not all right—it is a scandal—for a hospital mistakenly to mix up babies in a nursery. Parents do not want just to go home with a healthy baby; they want to go home with *their* baby, healthy or not. The questions to ask in this context are just why we accord the biological relationship value and whether we have good reason to do so.

To reiterate, I think that Lauritzen is right that: "while genetic connection may foster relational bonds, it is the bonds that are crucial, not the genetic ties."[81] But the fact that many adopted persons who already have all the genetic information that they want, and also know why their birth parents relinquished them, search for these parents nonetheless ought to give us pause. An adopted person may well enjoy the most secure and happy of relationships with his or her adoptive parents, yet long to know his or her birth parents and feel a profound sense of loss over not having relationships with these parents in his or her life. From this perspective, it seems, so-called responsible child "abandonment" just is not responsible enough.[82]

What it is blind to, I think, is the fact that, similarly to how a child whom one has lost cannot simply be replaced and made up for by a new child, even if that new child turns out to be wonderful in many ways (let us say—absurdly—"better" than the child who was lost),[83] a parent whom one has not known cannot simply be replaced and made up for by a parent who has made one his or her own. In other words, the loss of the relationship with one's birth parents cannot be *eliminated* by having a loving relationship with adoptive parents. We can acknowledge that a loving relationship with adoptive parents is a great good, and we can recognize that it may well provide consolation; but a unique relationship, because it is a relationship with persons to whom one is uniquely bound (flesh of flesh, bone of bones), has nonetheless been lost. By way of analogy, imagine that one's spouse with whom one has a healthy, loving relationship decides to leave one, but offers the apology that there is another, in fact much better person eager and willing to take his or her place. Would there be no loss? Clearly there would be: namely, the loss of the relationship, which cannot simply be made up for, since it was a relationship with a particular person, which was itself one of the goods of the relationship.

And yet the argument still cannot be considered closed. For there is no denying that the relationship between spouses is also disanalogous to the relationship between birth parents and a child: to the point for present purposes, a healthy, loving relationship between spouses already is rich, whereas the relationship between birth parents and a child is but potentially rich. Why accord this relationship any value, then, before it apparently becomes . . . well, valuable? Why claim that birth parents may not cast it away as a thing of little or no value when, in fact, it appears not yet to have any value? To the claim that the given, biological relationship ought not to be treated as a thing of little or no value and that one must accordingly have some justification for "abandoning" one's child to the care of willing and competent others, it could be objected that there are many people with whom one might develop, for example, rich friendships, yet one is not obligated, for this reason, to seek to become friends with any of these people, even if they very much want and would benefit from this relationship themselves. And so the question arises: even acknowledging the special nature of the relationship between procreators and child, what reason is there to think that there is a prima facie, all-things-considered obligation for procreators to *develop* this relationship? This question bears not only on the ethics of adoption, but on the ethics of gamete donation and surrogacy, as we shall see.

In the end, return to the observation with which this chapter began: one of the things that parents do for children is to presume to bring them into being. This, surely, is no little thing to answer for. For what a presumption! Chapter 2 focuses on how one incurs parental obligations, or what I call there procreative costs, and just what these obligations or costs amount to. After elaborating this account, I circle back to the loose ends of this opening chapter's argument.

2 The Costs of Procreation

As I noted in the introduction, contemporary philosophy offers two main accounts of how parental obligations or responsibilities are acquired. (Following most of the literature on this question, I use the terms 'obligations' and 'responsibilities' interchangeably.[1]) One is the so-called causal account, according to which women and men acquire parental obligations to a child by voluntarily acting in such a way that the coming-into-being of this child was a reasonably foreseeable consequence in the normal course of events. The second account of how parental obligations are acquired is the so-called voluntarist account, according to which parental obligations are acquired only by voluntary assumption of these obligations. A voluntarist understanding of parental obligations was notoriously taken for granted by Judith Jarvis Thomson in her famous defense of abortion several decades ago, and contemporary voluntarists typically fly under her flag. "Surely," Thomson declared, "we do not have any 'special responsibility' for a person unless we have assumed it, explicitly or implicitly."[2] For Thomson, nonvoluntary role obligations do not exist—though it is worth remarking that filial obligations, which she does not consider, at least seem to tell a different story. In this case, it seems, voluntarism comes too late. For, arguably, a child is *born into* filial obligations, not simply by being begotten, but by being carried to birth, nurtured, educated, and in sum cared for, to the point that she is then capable of responsibly exercising her will and so voluntarily assuming special responsibilities to others. Arguably again, however, it is too late at this point for the child-become-adult to decide *against* incurring special responsibilities to her parents. For, by virtue of her parents' having raised her, the child-become-adult already has filial obligations, whether she then likes it or not. (I do not pretend, by the way, to have established this claim.[3] My point here is simply that Thomson's declaration is by no means self-evident.)

Whatever we are to think of the claim that *all* special obligations or responsibilities can be acquired only by voluntarily undertaking them, the claim that *parental* obligations can be acquired only in this way has lately won strong support, buttressed in part, it stands to reason, by the practices of gamete donation, surrogacy, and perhaps abortion. By contrast, the causal account of parental obligations has not fared well at the hands of philosophers in recent years. Notably, in two provocative and sharply argued papers, Elizabeth Brake has challenged the causal account on multiple grounds and defended and developed a thorough-going voluntarist alternative.

In the first of these two papers, "Fatherhood and Child Support: Do Men Have a Right to Choose?" Brake focuses on the relevance of abortion rights to parental obligations. She makes, in brief, an argument from precedent, drawing on Thomson's defense of abortion. (I examine this argument of Brake's in chapter 3.) In the second paper, "Willing Parents: A Voluntarist Account of Parental Role Obligations," Brake changes strategy. Here her argument develops from the observation, made against critics who claim that voluntarism warrants abandoning a child to his or her death, that "parental obligations differ from general duties of rescue."[4] Against such critics, Brake affirms that "[e]veryone in a position to save the life of a child has a (*prima facie*) duty to do so."[5] But the question to ask is whether a woman and a man who voluntarily have sex and together produce a child have thereby the full range of parental obligations to him or her as conventionally understood (I put aside whatever this understanding is supposed to be), or only some smaller set of duties, perhaps only a duty of rescue. Brake does not dispute that the woman and man, as the child's biological parents, likely have at least *some* responsibilities toward the child. What is subject to dispute is whether the fact that they brought the child into being renders the woman and man prima facie responsible for all the obligations of training the child up. In line with Thomson's declaration that "[s]urely we do not have any 'special responsibility' for a person unless we have assumed it, explicitly or implicitly,"[6] the voluntarist, of course, says no.

Brake once suggests this line of argumentation in "Fatherhood and Child Support"—"causal responsibility," she comments, "should not be confused with moral responsibility, nor moral responsibility with an obligation to bear all costs of one's actions"[7]—but there she focuses on the first of the two claims in this quotation and leaves the second undeveloped. "Willing Parents," by contrast, seeks to secure the claim that moral responsibility for a child at birth, what Brake calls procreative costs, should not be confused with long-term responsibilities for the child. Here, I think, she poses a formidable challenge to the causal account—and also indicates a way that the inquiry of chapter 1 into the obligations of procreators toward children might be developed, namely, by critically evaluating her reckoning of the costs of procreation (which is her terminology for the sum of obligations one incurs by bringing a child into being). My interest here, to be clear, is in these costs, and not in defending the claim that all parental obligations as conventionally understood can be vindicated by the causal account.

Several more introductory points are in order. First, a note about terminology: I use in the following Brake's language of the "costs of pro-creation" and "procreative costs" because it has the advantage of focusing attention on the sum of obligations one incurs by bringing a child into being—whether we would want to call the parties to this act parents or not (that is, whether the language of *parental* obligations seems to fit or not). Second, Brake is not, of course, the only author who has challenged the claim that procreation gives rise to prima facie parental obligations. The literature on procreation and parenting is already large and lately growing. By way of example, David Archard has written in support of the causal account, but claimed that causing a child to exist does not obligate one to rear that child.[8] For Archard, the obligation that one incurs by causing a child to exist is to see to it that someone acts as his or her parent, not necessarily to do so oneself. (It is Archard who defends "the permissibility under some circumstances of child abandonment,"[9] discussed toward the end of my chapter 1.) I respond to Archard and others in the course of this chapter and the next two, but my focus here is Brake, whose thinking I use as a foil to develop my own. I focus on Brake because she is not afraid to follow the logic of voluntarism to its end.

The third point is related: in replying to Brake's challenge, I do not then pretend to counter all possible objections to the causal account, which is vulnerable on other grounds as well. Again by way of example, a com-mon charge leveled against the causal account is that many people may hold responsibility for the existence of a child, among others "biological and commissioning parents, grand-parents, matchmakers, doctors and lab technicians, pro-natalist friends."[10] So how nonarbitrarily to determine, on its grounds, who counts as a proximate (or "material" or "substan-tial") cause among what Giuliana Fuscaldo has termed "the countless contributing factors" leading to a child's existence?[11] To use the example that Fuscaldo gives, in an IVF (in vitro fertilization) pregnancy, is the prox-imate cause of the coming-into-being of the child "the action of the man and woman who provide the gametes, the embryologist who inseminates the egg, [or] the clinician who performs the embryo transfer, and so on?"[12] Each of these parties has a claim to being a necessary part of a suffi-cient condition for the child's coming-into-being, but it is unlikely that we would want to call the embryologist and clinician parents of the child and say that they bear parental obligations. Why not is another matter. The claim that they are not proximate causes of the child's coming-into-being appears vulnerable to the charge that our account of causation has been rigged for the purpose of delivering the answer that we want: that embry-ologists and clinicians, as well as brokers and lawyers, bear no parental obligations or responsibilities, despite the pivotal roles they may play in bringing a child into being. In brief, I am well aware of this challenge to the causal account—but addressing it is the work of chapter 4, not chapter 2. Here my question is simply this: what are the costs of procreation?

§1. RECKONINGS

To reiterate, according to the causal account of parental obligations or responsibilities, women and men incur parental obligations to a child by voluntarily acting in such a way that the coming-into-being of this child was a reasonably foreseeable consequence in the normal course of events. Consider the following example. Jeffrey Blustein presents the case of two persons, Joan and Anthony, who have sex using contraceptives. "Despite having taken reasonable care to avoid conception, Joan becomes pregnant," and decides neither to have an abortion nor to give up the child for adoption. Instead, "she reluctantly contacts Anthony," from whom she has since separated, and asks him to contribute toward the child's upbringing, since after all he not only is the child's biological father, but more to the point he voluntarily had sex with Joan and not only pregnancy, but the birth of a child are reasonably foreseeable risks of sex even with the use of contraceptives.[13] According to Blustein, that Anthony voluntarily had sex, and so participated in the creation of a being who will be harmed if it is not protected, means that he incurs "at least a prima facie obligation to *prevent* harm from coming" to the child or, positively stated, an obligation "to care for the child that is born" such that he or she may have reasonable assurance of a minimally decent life.[14] Yes, Anthony did not choose to procreate, and Joan had a choice that he did not have, namely, whether to terminate the pregnancy; but Blustein counters that Anthony did have "some control over becoming a parent," namely, his "choice whether to engage in risky activity." That he chose to engage in it and that a child resulted means that he has parental responsibilities, not because he *chose* to seek to become a father, but simply because having sex is a high-risk action for which one incurs strict liability on the condition that it is voluntarily done.[15] (Readers might wonder whether Blustein is warranted in dismissing the relevance of abortion rights to the question of the father's obligations to the child, but I put aside this concern until chapter 3.)

By contrast, according to Brake's "Willing Parents,"

1. Special obligations only arise through voluntary undertaking or as compensation for some harm.
2. Parental obligations are special obligations.
3. Thus, parental obligations are either the result of voluntary undertaking or else owed as compensation for some harm done to the child. (1, 2)
4. Parental obligations are not compensatory obligations.
5. Parental obligations arise through voluntary undertaking. (3, 4)[16]

The first premise is open to the immediate objection that there at least appear to be some special obligations—for example, filial obligations, or perhaps the obligations of citizenship—that arise neither through voluntary undertaking, nor as compensation for some harm, but arise nonetheless. (By special obligations, understand "obligations that are owed not to all persons, but to some limited class of persons, where the fundamental justification for the having of such obligations is not the intrinsic nature of the obligee as such," but instead or at least also the relation in which one stands toward the obligee.[17]) Michael Hardimon has distinguished two sorts of role obligations: what he calls contractual and noncontractual. The first sort we choose or "sign onto," whether by "a discrete, punctual act" like taking an oath of office, or "gradually, in a step-by-step way," such that acceptance of the social role is tacit, though normally no less clear than acceptance of the roles of, say, public official or spouse.[18] The second sort of role obligations, namely, the noncontractual, we neither sign onto, nor are impressed into against our will "like the seamen of old."[19] Instead, these are role obligations, like those of son or daughter, brother or sister, and perhaps citizen, "into which we are born."[20]

Brake anticipates this objection, and in the end more or less concedes it. For she replies by distinguishing one class of special obligations—namely, parental obligations—from another—among which filial obligations— and claiming that the former but not the latter arise only through voluntary undertaking or as compensation for some harm. According to Brake, as "we are not born into parental roles" but "can only take [these roles] on later in life,"[21] parental role obligations must *not* be noncontractual in the way that filial obligations at least appear to be. It might be countered, however, that parents are "born into" parental obligations in a different sense: that they are *carried into* these obligations, not involuntarily "like the seamen of old," but by virtue of having voluntarily engaged in actions that had the reasonably foreseeable consequence of bringing a child into existence in the normal course of events. And proponents of the causal account say, of course, just this.

Brake's argument really begins, then, with her third premise. This premise reads, to recall, that "parental obligations are either the result of voluntary undertaking or else owed as compensation for some harm done to the child." The second alternative is apparently supposed to represent the causal account. That compensation is "owed . . . for some harm done to the child" is not quite, however, what proponents of the causal account like Blustein say. More precisely, they say, not that a child has been harmed by having been brought into existence in a needy condition, but that the persons causally responsible for bringing the child into existence in this condition bear moral responsibility to *prevent* harm from coming to the child and to ensure that he or she has reasonable assurance of a minimally decent life.[22] Brake construes these obligations as "compensatory" and claims that "viewing parental obligations as compensatory reflects an impoverished conception of parenting."[23] In other words, according to her, "there is an explanatory gap between compensatory obligations, or 'procreative costs,' and moral parental obligations," such that having the former does not translate into having the latter.[24]

That "compensation" is not quite the right notion here can be appreciated by quoting Brake herself further. As she observes, "The classic doctrine of compensation is that the victim of harm be made whole—that is, restored to her unharmed state or the state she would have been in had the harm not occurred." Yet "an infant's needy state cannot be disentangled from its existence," and so "restoring the child to its prior state" makes no sense—unless we were to think of infanticide as a form of compensation, which is nonsense again.[25] The conclusion that should be drawn, it seems, is that it does not then make sense to conceive of so-called procreative costs as compensatory—but Brake does not draw this conclusion, instead persisting in speaking of the child as being in a "harmed state" for which procreators bear causal and moral responsibility. Given that an infant's needy state cannot be disentangled from its existence, "at best," Brake writes, "procreators can remove the child from its harmed state by bringing it to a less needy condition."[26] This is all the "compensation" that they can be claimed to owe.

Brake's argumentative strategy should be evident already: it is to concede, at least for the sake of argument, that the causal account is right that "causing a child to exist (given that the agent acted freely and that the effect was reasonably foreseeable) entails moral responsibility for the child's existence,"[27] but then to stress the gap between the purportedly compensatory obligations that a person thereby incurs and parental obligations as conventionally understood (which is her premise 4). What must fill in this gap, for her, is "voluntarily accepting the social and legal role of parent," which she presents as "necessary for moral parenthood" (her conclusion, step 5).[28] I think that it is at least disputable, however, whether procreative costs ought to be conceived as compensatory. As, according to the causal account presented by Blustein, an infant has not been harmed by having been brought into existence, but put at risk of harm, what is called for is not compensation, but care lest harm come the infant's way. Yet, in the end, I also think that Brake's basic point stands. For *if*, on the causal account, what procreators are responsible for is to prevent harm from coming to a child and to ensure that he or she has reasonable assurance of a minimally decent life (which is what Blustein says),[29] then "these procreative costs are not equivalent to parental obligations, at least as construed, for example, in the contemporary U.S."[30] In other words, the gap remains. As Brake remarks:

Contemporary parental obligations are extraordinarily weighty in duration and scope. . . . Legally, for example, parents are responsible for a much longer period than mere survival requires. . . . Socially, not only are parents expected to provide [at least] eighteen years of support, warmth, and affection, they are expected to enrich children's lives and enable them to flourish. These expectations are all to the best; but they entail that parental obligations exceed procreative costs.[31]

In sum, while "[s]ome contemporary parental obligations—such as providing healthcare or nutrition—can be explained as procreative costs," yet "others—long-term support obligations, warmth, and intimacy—exceed such procreative costs, *if* those are set at what is needed to repair a child's neediness and enable it to live a minimally decent life" (emphasis added).[32]

§2. ANOTHER ACCOUNT

Since contemporary proponents of the causal account typically *do* set so-called procreative costs more or less at what is needed to repair a child's neediness and to enable the child to live a decent life, the case for the voluntarist account of parental obligations might be considered clinched. An earlier, quite distinguished proponent of the causal account, however, set the procreative costs differently, and so we need to consider this variation. According to Kant, it is a "quite correct and even necessary idea to regard the act of procreation as one through which a person has been placed into the world without his consent and brought into it through no determination of his own, for which deed the parents incur an obligation to make [the person] content with his condition so far as they can."[33] Note that the focus here is not on the child's neediness and vulnerability to harm; instead, it is on the fact that a child is "placed into the world without his consent." From this starting point, Kant accordingly claims not merely that parents, qua procreators, must see to it that the child is not harmed, but that they must see to it that the child is made "content with his condition so far as they can"—however we understand it, a very high demand.

It might be countered, however, that this demand is even absurdly high. For surely the obligation to seek to make a child "content with his condition" extends well beyond what people normally think about parental obligations. It seems absurd to claim that parents, qua procreators, have an obligation to seek to provide a child—grown or not—with whatever it would take (within only the bounds of morality) to make the child content with having been brought into being. I think that this objection is right, but surely it is wrong that "what people normally think about parental obligations," to appeal to the same standard that the objection does, extends *only* to repairing a child's neediness and enabling him or her to live a minimally decent life. By contrast, Locke ascribed to children "a right not only to a bare Subsistence [*sic*] but to the comforts and conveniences of Life, as far as the conditions of their Parents can afford it";[34] and it is generally agreed that at least we moderns in the industrialized West count as "Locke's children" with respect to our thinking about the parent-child relationship.[35]

The claim that parents have an obligation to provide children "the comforts and conveniences of Life" is vulnerable, however, to the same objection as the claim that parents, qua procreators, have an obligation to seek to make a child "content with his condition": in brief, both claim too much. According to Joseph Millum, "were parental obligations the product of causing the existence of a person with needs, it should be legitimate for an adult to demand that her parents support her, even if she could do it herself."[36] But, Millum goes on, this claim (that it should be legitimate, etc.) conflicts with the belief that "the extent of parental responsibilities diminishes as the child grows older and more independent."[37] And so, assuming that this belief is not open to revision, parental obligations must *not* result from causing the existence of a person. In other words, the causal account must be wrong. If Kant's variation of the causal account is to have any plausibility, we need some way to counter this objection. So we need to think again about what obligations, if any, procreators incur by bringing a child unbidden into being.

The question has received more attention in literature than in philosophy. Recall Adam's outburst to God quoted in chapter 1:

"Did I request Thee, Maker, from my clay
To mold me Man? Did I solicit Thee
From darkness to promote me . . .?"[38]

Coming from an adolescent angry with his or her parents for some or other exercise of parental authority, such a complaint—duly reformulated!—would be difficult to take seriously. The complaint is likewise dubious coming from Milton's Adam, as he himself goes on to recognize. Before Adam's act of disobedience, God had tended to his every need. "[W]ilt thou enjoy the good, /Then cavil the conditions?" Adam accordingly asks himself, considering what he would make of such a complaint—"Wherefore didst thou beget me? I sought it not!"—should it be made by a son of his angry over the punishment for an act of disobedience.[39] In any event, Adam's question, "[W]ilt thou enjoy the good, /Then cavil the conditions?" is worth examining. It might be understood as implying that bringing a child unbidden into being is justifiable inasmuch as life—simply the gift of life itself—is a good, whatever its conditions. Or it might be understood as implying that bringing a child unbidden into being is justifiable inasmuch as the child is given a good life—more precisely, inasmuch as procreators do what they can to give the child a good life—which is to say one that the child has reason to affirm, even if he or she does not in fact affirm it.

The difference is significant. Against the background of a life that has known love and care as well as some measure of "comforts and conveniences," Adam's complaint is dubious coming from him and difficult to take seriously coming from the angry adolescent; but it would be much more credible coming from Victor Frankenstein's nameless creature (recall that Shelley uses Adam's outburst as her novel's epigraph), abandoned at his "birth" to his own devices, condemned by his ghoulish looks and terrifying size to a life alienated from all human society and sympathies. Frankenstein's creature seems justified in claiming that Victor *owes* him for having brought him unbidden into being, which is to say that the gift of life was not gift enough.[40] (Here the notion of compensation reenters the equation.) Moreover, Frankenstein's creature seems justified in claiming that Victor wronged him, not only by abandoning him and thereby depriving him of self-knowledge and family,[41] but by having brought him into being in the condition that he is, "with a figure hideously deformed and loathsome."[42] Just what Victor owes the creature, however, is another question. Victor seems right in reneging on his promise to make the creature a female companion—after all, could her consent to this arrangement be presumed?[43]—but his agonizing over the right course of action only underscores the irresponsibility of his bringing the creature into being to begin with.

Shelley's novel thus not only supports the intuition that a procreator incurs a responsibility to make his or her child "content with his condition" (problematic though this language is), but suggests a reason why. In brief, the gift of life may be a burden and, in extreme cases, even a curse. Recall as well Job's great cry from the heart:

> Let the day perish in which I
> was born.
> and the night that said,
> "A man-child is conceived."
> Let that day be darkness!
> May God above not seek it,
> or light shine on it.
> Let gloom and deep darkness
> claim it.[44]

Of course, there is nothing that Job's *parents* could have done to save Job from his suffering, other than not have brought him into being, in which case there would not even have been a Job to protect. But there is much that parents can do to strive to avert suffering in a child's life once he or she is in existence, and perhaps much that they ought to do, morally, to reconcile a child to, and to fortify him or her for, the inevitable trials and ills of life, among which the terror of death. If life is not an unequivocal good, then procreation is not a morally innocent undertaking, and it makes sense to think that a procreator has much to answer for in bringing a child unbidden into being.

Philosophers have given much attention to the puzzles of wrongful life and wrongful disability, but comparatively little to the question of

whether procreation without such complications is at all morally problematic or at least ambivalent. We do, however, have one searching
account of this question, namely, Seana Valentine Shiffrin's "Wrongful
Life, Procreative Responsibility, and the Significance of Harm," and this
account can help make my considerations so far more rigorous and move
us beyond intuitions.[45]

Recall my two interpretations of Adam's question, "[W]ilt thou enjoy
the good, /Then cavil the conditions?" First, the question might be understood as implying that bringing a child unbidden into being is justifiable
inasmuch as life—simply the gift of life itself—is a good, whatever its
conditions.[46] Or it might be understood as implying that bringing a child
unbidden into being is justifiable inasmuch as the child is given a good
life—more precisely, inasmuch as procreators do what they can to give
the child a good life—which is to say one that the child has reason to
affirm. Shiffrin argues strongly for the second line of thought. Her basic
thesis is that procreation "faces difficult justificatory hurdles because it
involves imposing serious harms and risks on someone who is not in
danger of suffering greater harm if one does not act," since otherwise the
person would simply not come into being.[47] Yes, for sure, life can be a
great good, for which gratitude to one's parents, or the gods or God, is
the appropriate response; but it should not be pretended that life is easy,
or forgotten that it can prove trying and even excruciating. By being
caused to exist, children are thrown into a drama the denouement of
which is death. Along the way, they can expect to suffer loss; undergo
significant disappointment; be subject to anxiety, distress, and even terror; be afflicted with sickness and pain (even terrible, debilitating pain);
and face wrenching moral questions and quandaries. They are also made
vulnerable to risks taken by procreators, risks that may render life a trial
or worse even from the beginning.[48] Frankenstein's creature serves in this
regard as a simple literary example.

The critical point here is that "[a]ll these burdens are imposed without
the future child's consent."[49] As David Velleman has nicely remarked,
"The opportunity wrapped up in the gift of life is thus an offer of the sort
that the child cannot refuse."[50] Moreover, appeal to hypothetical consent
is problematic for four reasons: (1) the fact that "great harm is not at stake
if no action is taken"; (2) the fact that, "if the action is taken, the harms
suffered may be severe"; (3) the fact that "the imposed action cannot be
escaped without high costs," namely, the physical, emotional, and moral
suffering of suicide; and (4) the fact that the hypothetical consent cannot
be "based on features of the individual who will bear the imposed condition," since that individual, not yet existing, is not yet known.[51]

The conclusion is not difficult to draw: since procreation imposes
such burdens and risks on the resulting child without his or her consent,
procreators have, at the least, responsibilities to avert the risks, where
possible, and to help the child bear the inevitable burdens.[52] In other

words, procreators have obligations extending well beyond ensuring that the child has a mere "life worth living," which is to say a life that would *not* inspire the judgment that it would have been a mercy had the child not been born.[53] Yet there is more. On this account, procreators also have obligations extending well beyond repairing a child's neediness and enabling him or her to live a minimally decent life—well beyond, that is, Brake's reckoning of the costs of procreation.

I think we can now speak more concretely about procreators' obligations. Preventing harm by providing or arranging for the provision of care during childhood is clearly a prima facie duty that procreators incur. (I roughly observe here Kant's distinction between duty and obligation: duty is "the matter of obligation," which is to say that which a person is bound to do by reason of being under an obligation.[54]) So too, to the end of preventing harm as well as to that of preparing a child for a decent life, is providing or in any event arranging for financial support during a child's minority. These duties appear to fall within Brake's reckoning of the costs of procreation. Yet preventing harm and securing financial support are by no means all that is called for. For children also require emotional support in the face of life's burdens and travails, which is another need that procreators are responsible for creating in presuming to bring children into being. And so procreators have, as well, a prima facie duty to see to it that these children enjoy deep, loving parent-child relationships, as it is just such relationships that fortify children for and begin to reconcile them to life's trials. Now, no doubt persons other than one's parents can help one come to terms with life, and admittedly this is work that we all must do by ourselves throughout our lives; but parents (whether procreators or not) have the critical responsibility to give us the intellectual, emotional, cultural, and perhaps as well spiritual tools to this end, to foster in us the resolve, and to help us on our way through the gift of a loving parent-child relationship with all its special goods, listed in chapter 1.

This last point calls for elaboration, not least because it allows us to return, at last, to the question with which chapter 1 concluded. Even acknowledging the special nature of the relationship between procreators and child (in a word, its "givenness"), what reason is there to think that there is a prima facie, all-things-considered obligation for procreators to *develop* this relationship? Recall that I raised there the objection that there are many people with whom one might develop rich friendships, yet one is not obligated, for this reason, to seek to become friends with any of these people. We can now say that the simple difference between these two cases is that one owes nothing to potential friends, whereas one has incurred great responsibilities to a child whom one has presumed to bring into being. To the point for present purposes, these responsibilities include answering for what one has presumed to do, which obviously one can do only *in person*, meaning which one cannot transfer to others who did not themselves bring the child into being.

Now, it might be claimed that, even so, the procreator is not him or herself obligated to be the one offering the child the love that he or she needs. Instead, what is nontransferrable is the obligation to see to it that *someone* loves the child as a parent. In other words, on this account (which should remind us of the transfer principle discussed in chapter 1), what the procreator cannot transfer to others is precisely, and only, the responsibility to *arrange* that the child has what he or she needs. So long as some willing, competent other is found, the procreator has done his or her duty, and has no further need to justify the "abandonment" of parental obligations (such as that he or she is incapable of carrying out these obligations). But this account will not do. The reason is that it fails to appreciate that, while no doubt persons other than one's *procreators* can help one come to terms with life (for example, adoptive parents), no one other than one's procreators—with the possible exception of the Creator—can be called on to answer for the fact of one's being. No one else, that is, has or can even assume this charge. As Shiffrin has observed, deep parent-child relationships may reconcile a child to the fact and conditions of his or her existence, and make the child's life one that he or she has reason to affirm, in part because they "permit children to confront, hold responsible, show gratitude toward, and receive comfort and instruction from *those who have given them this burden-riddled mixed benefit*"—which of course only procreators did.[55]

Take again Frankenstein's creature. Say, to vary Shelley's story, Frankenstein had found for the creature a loving adoptive parent whom Frankenstein had "good reason" to believe would faithfully carry out the obligations of parenthood by doing what he or she could to prevent harm from coming the creature's way, by preparing the creature for a decent life, and by cultivating with him a deep parent-child relationship that would fortify him for and go some ways toward reconciling him to the travails and burdens of life. Would Frankenstein then be free and clear from all obligations to the creature? In particular, if in later years the creature wanted to meet with Frankenstein, to speak with him, to come to know him, indeed to have a relationship with him, out of a felt need (however vaguely articulated) to come to terms with this life that Frankenstein had presumed to give him, would Frankenstein be warranted in saying no, on the grounds that he had already done all his duties toward the creature by finding him the loving adoptive parent? I think that the answer to this question is itself clearly *no*, that Frankenstein would *not* be warranted in saying no to the creature *on these grounds*.[56] For it was Frankenstein, not the adoptive parent, who gave the creature the "burden-riddled mixed benefit" of life, for which he then has an obligation to answer, as best he can, should the creature come to him in a time of need. (By the way, I say more on this point come chapter 4, in discussing the responsibilities of gamete providers and surrogates.)

It is, of course, a further question whether Frankenstein was justified *to begin with* in "abandoning" the creature to the loving adoptive parent.

To repeat from chapter 1, It is surely correct that a parent who with good reason does not believe him or herself capable of meeting parental obligations does right in surrendering her child to willing and competent others. As I stated there, this act can in fact be seen as "the last in a series of actions meant to provide care for the child."[57] But let us say that Frankenstein did not consider himself so incapable and had no good reason to hold otherwise. Was Frankenstein then justified in entrusting someone else to form a loving parent-child relationship with the creature?

I think that the answer is again no. I have argued in this chapter that the obligation to see to it that a child has a loving parent-child relationship in his or her life springs from the child's need (created by his or her procreators in creating the child, which they need not have done) for emotional support in the face of life's burdens: more fully, the child's need to be fortified against, prepared for, and reconciled to life's burdens and travails. To be sure, this need can be and very often is satisfied by adoptive parents, for which they deserve gratitude and recognition. But we do well here to recall the fact, cited in chapter 1, that many adopted persons who already have all the genetic information that they want, and know why their birth parents relinquished them, and enjoy secure and happy relationships with their adoptive parents, search for their birth parents nonetheless. This fact indicates that, at least within the world we know with its kinship structures, the child's need for emotional support is answered most adequately—and so we could say answered most *responsibly*—by a relationship with his or her biological procreators (in the following sentences, I say simply "procreators"). It is clearly better that procreators be responsible to the child later in his or her life than not at all. But data about adopted persons' experiences suggest that it would be better yet—and more responsible yet—for procreators to be present to the child throughout his or her life. Accordingly, procreators have a prima facie, all-things-considered obligation to develop loving parent-relationships with the children whom they presume to bring into being, during these children's minority and beyond— the conclusion for which chapter 1 long sought.[58] (To reiterate, calling this obligation prima facie means that it may in some circumstances be overridden—another point to which chapter 4 returns.)

What is wrong with Millum's objection that "were parental responsibilities the product of causing the existence of a person with needs, it should be legitimate for an adult to demand that her parents support her, even if she could do it herself,"[59] is that the needs of a grown child who is competent to take care of herself are not needs that her parents concomitantly caused in causing her existence. A person whom I injured in some way in the course of a high-risk action like driving has needs that I caused in injuring her. I am, then, morally responsible for those needs, but only those needs and not others that I did not cause. Likewise, young children have needs for which parents bear responsibility in having caused these children to come into existence. To survive and to be prepared to live decent lives, they need, among other things, food, clothing, shelter, medical care, and education. To come to terms with life's burdens and travails, they need, in brief, love, as well as culture and perhaps some form of spirituality. These are all needs that the parents caused in bringing the child into being. Now, a competent grown child may need, for example, money to buy a car; but this need is not one that parents concomitantly caused in causing the child to exist, and so it is not a need for which they are morally responsible. Instead, what the competent grown child needs to do here is to put to work the talents that his or her parents were obligated to help him or her cultivate. Even the grown child, however, has a prima facie justified claim on his or her parents to keep up and, if need be, reestablish the parent-child relationship. For this relationship, so long as it is reasonably healthy and not toxic for any of the parties, may provide special goods, like unconditional love, abiding interest, and deep-rooted concern, which can hardly be had from anyone other than one's parents and that, if they are had, make life much less forbidding than it would otherwise be.[60] Positively stated, these goods can help reconcile one to existence, a need that parents, qua procreators, do cause and that adoptive parents, in assuming the obligations of birth parents, take responsibility for to the extent that they can.

Against this background, the contemporary focus on preventing harm cannot but appear as strikingly narrow, and the corresponding assessment of procreative costs as all too low. On the account that this chapter has developed, by bringing a child unbidden into being, a procreator acquires the prima facie obligations, not only to prevent harm and to prepare the child for a decent life, but to provide, *in person*, support, warmth, and affection during the child's minority and beyond—that is, to develop a loving parent-child relationship with him or her. Lest my argument be misunderstood, I have not denied that the obligations incurred by procreators may, in some circumstances, rightly be transferred to others (though adoptive parents cannot answer, as procreators can, for the child's having been brought into being). I also have not claimed that parents, whether biological or adoptive, must suffer lovingly at the hands of vicious grown children. To repeat from chapter 1, the pain of a thankless, or worse, older child may break the human heart.

§3. THE OFFICES OF NATURE[61]

One final objection of a different kind, however, has to be anticipated. Since Kant, the standard response to the biblical commandment to love has been that our affections are not ours to command, and so, according to the dictum that ought implies can, an obligation to develop a deep bond of affection with another cannot reasonably be demanded. In the poet Eugenio Montale's memorable phrase, the heart is a "discordant instrument" that will not always let itself be played.[62] The most that can be demanded, then, is what Kant called *amor benevolentiae*: benevolence or "practical love."[63] On this account, we must say that the parent who fails to love his or her child, and so to cultivate a deep loving relationship with him or her, has not violated any obligation toward that child.[64] Maybe we could say still that the parent is deficient somehow, but we could not characterize this deficiency as a moral failing.

To begin with, it might well be disputed whether Kant is right that we cannot bring ourselves to love another (using this emotion term non-episodically: when we say that we love someone, we are not referring to a distinct emotion-episode, as we are when we speak of feeling, for example, lust or envy toward someone).[65] As Alasdair MacIntyre has remarked, while in particular situations it may be true that we cannot command our feelings, it is no less true that we can "cultivate and train our dispositions to feel, just as we can train our dispositions to act and indeed our dispositions to act with and from certain feelings."[66] David Hume put the point this way:

> When any virtuous motive or principle is common in human nature, a person, who feels his heart devoid of that principle, may hate himself upon that account, and may perform the action without the motive, from a certain sense of duty, in order to acquire by practice, that virtuous principle, or at least, to disguise to himself, as much as possible, his want of it.[67]

Others have sketched out methods to "bring about particular emotions, including the emotional aspect of love."[68] These methods include giving ourselves reasons to feel this or that way, like "a boxer telling himself to become angry to prepare for a fight, or Tolstoy telling himself that he should feel grief, when attending his grandparent's funeral."[69] Another method is reflecting on the reasons why we feel this way or that, with the possibility of coming to feel differently if we find that our feelings are not supported by good reasons, like a mother-in-law changing her feelings toward her daughter-in-law after realizing that past feelings of contempt had been based on jealousy.[70] And finally we might "deliberately . . . place ourselves in situations in which we know that we would probably experience particular emotions," like piety at church, or compassion at a homeless shelter.[71]

There are, however, limits to our control of our feelings; the poet does not lie in picturing the heart as a "discordant instrument" that does not always let itself be played. Hume concedes as much in suggesting that a person whose heart is devoid of this or that natural affection—whose heart, in brief, is indisposed to love—may in the end simply have to disguise this want from himself. And another author who had claimed that we can choose "to embrace and cultivate the right feelings and motives" feels himself compelled to acknowledge in the end that, "[s]till, it is correct to say that [a duty of feeling] operates only within the limits of what we can control."[72] So Kant appears to be right in claiming that, if a person lacks endowments of feeling, or for whatever reason cannot bring his or her heart to feel this or that way, that person cannot rightly be criticized for violating a moral duty.

So it appears. But consider, by way of example, parents who attest to having no feeling for a child at birth and to having to learn to feel tenderness for him or her. Among these parents, some, faced with especially trying circumstances, even have to struggle heroically to train their hearts.[73] Yet not only does this struggle, if it is necessary, seem morally obligatory; it also seems morally obligatory for a parent to come out of this struggle victorious. The obverse of this claim is that a person who did not and could not come to develop a deep love for his or her child would have to be considered morally deficient. It is doubtful, in any event, that such a person could make much of a parent, which is to say parent well. Hume, whose thinking about morality appears at times diametrically opposed to Kant's, claims that "natural affection . . . is the duty of every parent" and that, "[w]ere natural affection not a duty, the care of children cou'd not be a duty," so much does this care presuppose and depend upon affection.[74] And Hume seems right here. The normative unconditionality of the parent-child relationship, which as I remarked in chapter 1 is of great importance for the child's sense of security and belonging as well as value, is founded on deep emotional attachment to the child on the part of the parent. As Onora O'Neill has remarked, "'good enough' parents usually accept not only the daily round of responsive parenting, but a view of their relationship to their children as long term, moreover as one that they will seek to sustain in the face of vicissitudes and difficulties that might destroy most relationships,"[75] in particular so-called chosen relationships like friendship or even marriage. To this end, love in a sense exceeding though not excluding benevolence appears indispensable. (Despite Kant's tendency to oppose benevolence and feeling, the duty of benevolence is perhaps best understood as the *form* that love should take, or to which it should conform. Love that is not informed by benevolence—in other words, love that not only exceeds benevolence, but also excludes it—risks harming rather than benefiting the beloved, as manic attachments and erotic infatuations might be called on to attest.[76])

The thought that a parent who did not and could not feel "natural affection" for his or her child would be morally wanting is, of course, alien to Kant's moral philosophy. For Kant, all that belongs to nature is unfree, and only the will, as free, is properly the object of moral assessment. Kant allows that there are "natural predispositions" that must be in place for the moral law to motivate us[77]—as another author has nicely put it, Kant rightly recognizes that "there can be no will to will things; [the will] needs a prior disposition . . . to provide a motive for acts of will,"[78]—but Kant denies that we can be accountable for, in his striking line, "the niggardly provision of a stepmother nature."[79] As Bernard Williams has characterized Kant's thinking here, "Anything which is the product of happy or unhappy contingency is no proper object of moral assessment"; even so-called constitutive luck—roughly, the luck of being this or that kind of person with this or that kind of heart—is put out of play.[80]

That we do not really believe this view—perhaps more precisely, that we do not live like it is true—can be realized, I think, if we consider how we would assess ourselves if we did not and could not deeply love our children, though this failing could not be imputed to our will. (Readers without children should imagine along. And again, I exclude vicious grown children.) Hume claims, as I have quoted him, that "a person, who feels his heart devoid of [any virtuous motive or principle that is common in human nature], may hate himself upon that account." Hate may seem too strong here, but regret does not seem strong enough. If we were this person, perhaps we would ask, with King Lear, what cause in nature there could be to make such a hard heart.[81] I imagine that we would lament, in other words, simply how we are.[82]

Whether we would be blameworthy is a further question. If our failing really could not be imputed to our will, I think that the answer must be no; but this answer supports the view, not that a failure to love cannot be a moral failing, but that, as Lawrence Blum suggested some time ago, the notions of blame and praise, and blameworthiness and praiseworthiness, "comprise only a subset of the concepts in terms of which we can be morally assessed and criticized."[83] The notion of blame seems closely connected with the will and moral agency; what Blum calls our "moral being" encompasses much more, including our attitudes toward others, our habits and patterns of sensitivity and compassion and empathy, and our moral imagination and vocabulary. Now, there is certainly a sense in which we would not be responsible for our hard hearts—what could we have done?—but the fact of our hard hearts (or racist hearts, or sexist hearts) would not excuse us from moral criticism. By way of example, others might criticize us, or we might criticize ourselves, for not having known better than to have wagered becoming parents in the first place.[84] For a parent who lacks affect toward his or her child is not a *good* parent. The lack of affect is a sign that he or she apparently does not see the good of having and caring for children, which someone who has children *ought* to see.[85] (By the way, while "natural affection" for one's child may be necessary for being a good parent, it should not be thought sufficient. A parent might have love for his or her child but be prevented from acting appropriately on that love by some internal or external constraint—for example, alcoholism.[86] In such a case, the parent would have the love, but fail to establish the deep loving relationship.)

To anticipate an objection, it might well be asked whether our so-called considered judgments on this matter should be considered sound. Appealing to these judgments, I have claimed that we believe "natural affection" to be a duty, but I have not, it might be observed, presented an argument, properly speaking, refuting Kant's view to the contrary. In response to this objection, it is worth noting that Kant's argument in the *Groundwork* for the claim that "the ground of obligation . . . must not be sought in the nature of the human being or in the circumstances of the world in which he is placed, but a priori simply in concepts of pure reason," itself appeals to "the common idea of duty and of moral laws." According to Kant, "Everyone must grant" that a moral law must hold not only for human beings, but for all rational beings. His example is the command, "Thou shalt not lie." It would be absurd to claim that other rational beings do not need to heed it, or in other words that what would be wrong for us to do might be right for other rational beings with different "empirical" natures from ours.[87] To which it makes sense to reply: yes, it does seem absurd to claim that what is wrong for us to do might be right for other, differently constituted rational beings; but it does *not* at all seem absurd to claim that other, differently constituted rational beings might not be enjoined to the same *positive* duties—for example, love of offspring, if angels (the standard philosophical example of other rational beings) could have any. In other words, it seems to make perfect sense to think that duties of virtue might well depend on the empirical "nature of the human being," and moreover might well make demands of it. And so I would say that the burden of proof to the contrary falls on Kant.[88] Kant is certainly right that we cannot bring ourselves to delight in another simply on command, but we can work to cultivate and secure a love for others that at once exceeds benevolence and runs deeper than mere *liking*.[89] To the point for present purposes, to develop a deep bond of affection with a child (not mere fleeting feelings, or for that matter "melting sympathy") may not be easy and may even demand a struggle; but that is a demand that morality, in the persons of our children, appears to make of our nature.

NOTE: THE CONVENTIONAL-ACTS ACCOUNT

It should be noted that contemporary philosophy offers a third account of how parental obligations or responsibilities are acquired, namely, Joseph Millum's "*conventional-acts* account, according to which parental duties are taken on by individuals through acts whose meaning is determined by social convention."[90] To reach this conclusion, Millum first distinguishes what he terms *natural duties*—"duties whose acquisition is independent of social conventions regarding their acquisition"—from what he terms *artificial duties*—"duties whose acquisition depends upon the existence of social conventions regarding their acquisition."[91] He then criticizes so-called natural duties accounts of the origins of parental responsibility and concludes, "by elimination," that parental duties "must be artificial."[92]

The present chapter has already countered some of Millum's criticisms of the causal account (in his terminology, a natural duties account); in the next two chapters, I have yet more to say in this regard. But here I offer a criticism in turn: Millum's "conventional-acts account" cannot, in the end, help us make headway in difficult cases. Consider his claim that "if an agent voluntarily (and knowingly) performs an act that others reasonably think is morally transformative . . ., it will have the transformative effect."[93] On what basis are others *reasonably* to think that the act is morally transformative? Is appeal to convention alone "reasonable" at this point? Or consider his claim that, on the conventional-acts account, "[a] woman has not taken on responsibility for a fetus through an act of intercourse, even if the fetus is a person, if either: there is not general agreement that the act of intercourse gives her this responsibility, or she reasonably thinks that she has not taken on responsibility in this way."[94] Should "general agreement"—without specification as to among whom and on what grounds—really be considered decisive here? The abortion debate is over precisely what our "conventions" *should* be—that is, what are the right "conventions" to have, such that the word 'conventions' is not quite right here. Further, to say that a woman has not taken on responsibility for a fetus through an act of intercourse if "she *reasonably* thinks that she has not taken on responsibility in this way" begs the question of what it is reasonable to think here, which surely is not just a matter of convention to which philosophical argumentation has nothing to contribute. In sum, appealing to convention finally raises more questions than it answers. What needs consideration is not merely what the social and legal "conventions" surrounding parenthood are, but what they *should* be.[95]

3 Abortion and the Grounds of Parental Obligations

Consider the following claim:

> Pregnancy, like disease transmission, is a proximate effect of sex; childbirth is determined by further steps, the woman's choice. While the father might be obligated to share the costs immediately incurred as a result of sex, his responsibility comes to an end when [the woman] gives birth. If the choice to bear and keep the child is solely the mother's, the *moral* responsibility for its existence seems to be hers alone.[1]

This claim is interesting in several respects. For one, it articulates what may someday become common sense.[2] Should abortion come to be seen as a morally neutral act, or carrying a child to term as merely morally permissible, it may come to be thought that *of course* it would be unfair to hold a man responsible for a woman's choice to carry a pregnancy to term when he would have chosen otherwise, should the choice have been his. The position that it would be unfair to hold the man responsible for the woman's choice clashes, however, with an intuition that it is mistaken to think that childbirth is not a "proximate effect" of sex, but the effect of an intervening action by the woman alone, namely, her having or not having an abortion. Surely, it might be countered, childbirth follows naturally not only from pregnancy, but from sex. And one is responsible for the consequences that follow, in the normal course of events, from one's actions, on the grounds that these consequences just are one's actions.

What else is interesting about the claim that I have quoted is that it casts as mere unsupported prejudice the belief that, all others things being equal, the fallback position in a pregnancy is to carry it to term.[3] Of course, this is a controversial claim in philosophical circles, but it seems right to say, as David Benatar does, that "most people tend to think that some reason needs to be provided *for* having or performing an abortion"—and I would venture that this statement holds even for most philosophers.[4] In other words, it is circumstances that may justify abortion, not pregnancy as such.[5] For the choice of whether or not to abort is not a choice between two morally equivalent options. Instead, on at least the generally prevailing view, given the goodness of human life, the choice is more heavily weighted toward going on with the pregnancy and becomes only more so as the pregnancy progresses.[6] Accordingly, it is *not* unfair to hold a man responsible for a child of his whom he would rather not have been born. For the man, by having voluntarily had sex, set in train a process that, once it is under way, there is good reason to carry to its natural end, namely, the birth of a child.

Perhaps not surprisingly given how provocative it is, the claim in question in the preceding paragraphs is Elizabeth Brake's. As I noted in the preceding chapter, Brake has written two papers against the causal account. "Willing Parents," which we examined in chapter 2, concedes, at least for the sake of argument, that procreators do incur some responsibilities—so-called procreative costs—by virtue of having voluntarily acted in such a way that the coming-into-being of a child was a reasonably foreseeable consequence in the normal course of events. Brake's thesis in that paper is that these procreative costs amount only to the responsibilities to prevent harm and to provide the child reasonable assurance of a minimally decent life—a reckoning of the costs of procreation that I have disputed as much too low. By contrast, Brake's other paper against the causal account, "Fatherhood and Child Support: Do Men Have a Right to Choose?" focuses on the relevance of abortion rights to parental obligations and takes a harder line. She makes, in brief, an argument from precedent, building on Judith Jarvis Thomson's defense of abortion. According to Brake, "if women's partial responsibility for pregnancy does not obligate them to support a fetus, then men's partial responsibility for pregnancy does not obligate them to support a resulting child,"[7] with the upshot that the fact that a woman and a man together caused this being is neither here nor there to the question of whether they bear parental responsibility for it.[8] More simply put, if a woman may morally choose to abort an unborn child, then a man who did not consent to become a father should have the right to choose not to parent the child—a right that, next to the woman's power over the child's life and death, might seem even modest by comparison (though it should not be overlooked that the choice not to parent the child might well have serious consequences for his or her life prospects). The director of the New York-based National Center for Men speaks in this regard, inelegantly, of a man's right to a "financial abortion."[9]

There is a measure of irony in Brake's drawing from Thomson in order to make the case that, given the moral permissibility of abortion, when the mother wants the child and the father does not, "*the father should bear no legal responsibility for the fetus-person either before or after birth*" and is at most morally responsible to make a good-faith offer to the woman to share the costs of securing an abortion.[10] Keith Pavlischek, whom I have just quoted, made just this argument some years ago—but with the goal, quite different from Brake's, of lending credence to the pro-life claims: first, "that an intimate connection exists between the way we collectively relate to the unborn and the way we relate to children after birth"; and, second, "that the abortion mentality simply reaffirms the worst historical failings, neglect, and chauvinism of males," a claim that he attributed to pro-life feminists.[11] Pavlischek thereby hoped "to force a dilemma on defenders of permissive abortion laws: either surrender the defense of abortion on demand . . ., or surrender the advocacy of paternal responsibility for children of mothers who choose to forego an abortion."[12] Whereas Pavlischek expected readers to deny the consequent (no paternal responsibility) and so, at the least, have to rethink the antecedent (abortion on demand), Brake, by contrast, replaces his modus tollens with a simple modus ponens.

The aim of the present chapter is to speak to the question, noted in passing in chapter 2, of the relevance of the fact that, when abortion is legal and available, a woman has a choice that a man does not, namely, whether or not to carry the pregnancy to term. To recall, in his example of Anthony and Joan, Blustein argues that a man who has sex with a woman incurs parental responsibilities should she carry the child to term, not because he *chose* to seek to become a father, but simply because having sex is a high-risk action for which one incurs strict liability on the condition that it is voluntarily done. I then noted that readers might wonder whether Blustein is warranted in dismissing the relevance of abortion rights to the question of the father's obligations to the child. This chapter seeks to defend Blustein's conclusion (and the causal account more generally) by rebutting Brake's argument from precedent.

To be clear, my primary interest is *not* in defending Thomson's argument (which is critical for Brake's) from the charge that it brings with it untoward consequences. In other words, I am not interested here in defending Thomson's defense of abortion—which instead I criticize extensively. But I also am not interested here in other arguments that could be made on different grounds for or against the moral permissibility of abortion: for example, arguments based on the moral standing of the fetus. Instead, my focus is on born children, not the unborn, and I do not then (*nota bene*: I do *not*) develop a position on whether women, or for that matter men, have parental obligations to children before birth (though it is an interesting and important question whether women have responsibilities to fetuses the women have decided to carry to term[13]). In brief, my interest lies in separating the question of the viability of the causal account from the question of the moral permissibility of abortion. Interestingly, Brake's claim that I quoted and discussed at the beginning of this chapter is not in fact central to her argument in "Fatherhood and Child Support." But the claim leaves little doubt that, for her, the viability of the causal account stands or falls with the permissibility of abortion.

§1. BRAKE AGAINST THE CAUSAL ACCOUNT

To review, on the causal account, consenting to or voluntarily assuming parental obligations is not always a necessary condition for acquiring them. Of course, in cases of adoption, when one has been deemed eligible to assume parental obligations and when the child in question is likewise eligible to be adopted, consenting to or voluntarily assuming parental obligations is both a necessary and a sufficient condition for acquiring them. But this fact hardly warrants the claim, made by Brake, that "the permissibility of adoption seems a decisive objection" against the causal account.[14] That voluntarily assuming parental obligations is necessary and sufficient for acquiring them in cases of adoption does not mean that voluntarily assuming them is necessary for acquiring them in all cases. More than respect for parsimony is needed to warrant the assumption that "moral parenthood is a unified phenomenon"—that is, that there is only one way for parental obligations to be acquired.[15] On the causal account, voluntarily acting in such a way that the coming-into-being of a child was a reasonably foreseeable consequence in the normal course of events is a sufficient condition for acquiring parental obligations to that child should he or she result. One need not have consented to these obligations, or even have consented to the birth of this child, as so-called unwilling fathers do not. (Unwilling fathers are men who voluntarily have sex with a woman, but unwillingly become fathers due to the decision of the woman not to have an abortion. A man may become an unwilling father because he and his partner did not use contraceptives, because the contraceptives failed, or because the woman misrepresented to him either that she was using contraceptives or that she would have an abortion should she become pregnant—all possibilities that a reasonable person would see as reasonably possible.) On the causal account, these men have parental obligations to the child by virtue of their causal role in the coming-into-being of the child, and *not* because consent to sex, given its risks even with contraceptives, allegedly implies tacit consent to parental obligations should a child be produced. (If consent is an attitude, then it makes little sense to say that persons consent to parental obligations simply by voluntarily having sex.[16]) One last time, what matters on the causal account is not that one voluntarily assumed or somehow consented to parental obligations, but that one is responsible for the reasonably foreseeable consequences of one's voluntary action—here, for the coming-into-being of a child. As James Nelson has succinctly put the point, on the causal account, "The content of our duties is not always a matter of our implicit decisions."[17]

As I have stated already, Brake's "Fatherhood and Child Support: Do Men Have a Right to Choose?" seeks to clear the way for the voluntarist account by focusing on the relevance of abortion rights to parental obligations. Again to reiterate, Brake makes an argument from precedent.

According to her, "if women's partial responsibility for pregnancy does not obligate them to support a fetus, then men's partial responsibility for pregnancy does not obligate them to support a resulting child,"[18] with the upshot that the fact that a woman and a man together caused this being is neither here nor there to the question of whether they bear responsibility for it.

It is important to note that this argument can work only if a fetus and a child have the same or at least relevantly similar moral standing: in other words, only if each deserves the same or at least relevantly similar consideration from its procreators. If a fetus deserved *less* consideration than a child, the fact that a woman would not be obligated to carry a fetus to term would have no immediate bearing on the question of a man's responsibility to the resulting child should the woman go through with the pregnancy. In other words (and the point is important, so worth repeating), if a fetus deserved *less* consideration than a child—in brief, if a fetus were *not* a person the same as a child, and so if a woman carrying a fetus stood in an essentially different relationship to it from that of a man to his child: she would be, strictly, a potential mother, he already a father—then the permissibility of abortion would be irrelevant to the question of the father's responsibilities. That is, it would be baseless for us to conclude that, as the woman is permitted to abort the fetus and so must not have parental obligations to it just by virtue of having coproduced it (the fetus), he too must not have parental obligations just by virtue of having coproduced him or her (the child). It makes sense, then, that to make her case Brake draws from Thomson's defense of abortion. For, as is well known, Thomson's paper grants, for the sake of argument, that the fetus is a person with the same moral standing as a child, but claims nonetheless that the conclusion that abortion is morally impermissible does not follow.[19]

It might be objected that, if women do not acquire parental obligations by having sex, then neither should men, whatever the standing of the fetus—thereby allowing us to bypass the complications of Thomson's defense. The causal account does not hold, however, that women or men acquire parental obligations by having sex. Instead, according to the causal account, they acquire parental obligations by bringing a child into being. For present purposes, I do not take a position on whether this remarkable event happens at some point before birth, and so I am perfectly willing to allow (again at least for present purposes) that fathers have parental obligations if and only if women carry the child to term.[20] My focus, to reiterate, is on born children, not the unborn. If the claim is to be made that an unwilling father does not bear responsibility for his child by virtue of having coproduced it, because the mother did not incur responsibility for the fetus by her role in its coproduction, the evidence for which is that she was within her rights to abort it, this evidence is relevant only if the child and the fetus have the same or at least relevantly similar moral standing. Otherwise, that a woman is within her rights to disclaim parental obligations to the fetus (by aborting it) is irrelevant to the question of whether a man is within his rights to disclaim parental obligations to the child (by refusing all procreative costs). So Thomson's defense of the moral permissibility of abortion, even granting the fetus full moral standing of a person, must be central to the case for unwilling fathers' own, more limited "right to choose."

Brake draws in particular on Thomson's counterexample to "the principle," as Brake terms it, "that we are morally responsible for *all* the foreseeable consequences of our actions."[21] Thomson famously asks us to imagine that

> people-seeds drift about in the air like pollen, and if you open your windows, one may drift in and take root in your carpets or upholstery. You don't want children, so you fix up your windows with fine mesh screens, the very best you can buy. As can happen, however, and on very, very rare occasions does happen, one of the screens is defective; and a seed drifts in and takes root.[22]

Thomson then asks: "Does the person-plant who now develops have a right to the use of your house?" And her answer is: "Surely not—despite the fact that you voluntarily opened your windows, you knowingly kept carpets or upholstered furniture, and you knew that screens were sometimes defective."[23] The conclusion that we are supposed to draw is that, just as it would be morally permissible to uproot a person-plant from one's house, so it would be morally permissible to expel a fetus, even if it has the full moral standing of a person, from one's uterus.

How Brake's argument unfolds from here is relatively simple. If we grant, at least for the sake of argument, that a fetus is a person with full moral standing (premise 1), and if we grant, presumably not only for the sake of argument, that a child is likewise a person (premise 2), then if it is the case that a woman is not obligated to support—that is, carry to term— a fetus just by virtue of having acted in such a way as to have caused its existence (premise 3, derived from Thomson's paper), it must also be the case that a man is not obligated to support—that is, provide for—the fetus-become-a-child (these are only different phases of the same person, not different substances) just by virtue of having acted in such a way as to have caused its existence (Brake's conclusion).[24] As Brake notes, by these lights, "the conception of parental responsibility underlying strict child support law comports uneasily with unrestricted legal access to abortion."[25] Moreover, by these lights, the causal account of parental obligations or responsibility must be false. For "[o]n [Thomson's] view," Brake writes in agreement, both fetuses and infants "gain rights against their parents when their parents voluntarily assume responsibility for them and not as a result of parents' causal responsibility for their conception."[26]

Brake certainly appears to have Thomson right here, though inter-estingly Thomson nowhere in her paper reflects on how men acquire parental obligations. The only remark in her paper that has any bearing on this question is that

> [i]f a set of parents do not try to prevent pregnancy, or do not obtain an abortion, and then at the time of the birth of the child do not put it out for adoption, but rather take it home with them, then they have assumed responsibility for it, they have given it rights, and they can-not *now* withdraw support from it at the cost of its life because they now find it difficult to go on providing for it.[27]

This remark seems, however, quite poorly considered. On what may be an uncharitable reading, it appears to sanction, before the moment of tak-ing the child home, simply abandoning a child and letting him or her die should providing for the child be found "difficult." But read charitably or not, Thomson does not say and gives us no means to determine *just how difficult* providing for the child must be found in order to justify "withdraw[ing] support from it at the cost of its life"—which is, to say the least, a significant oversight on her part.[28] Further, even if the "set of parents" do not have special, parental responsibilities to the child by vir-tue of having caused his or her coming-into-being, they nonetheless have a general duty of beneficence, here more precisely rescue, toward him or her, whether they have "given" the child rights or not. The question of rights is in fact irrelevant in this regard; what matters is the parents' obligations, which need not correspond to any rights on the part of the child, as so-called imperfect obligations do not.

A voluntarist account of parental obligations need not, however, deny that it would be wrong to abandon a child to death. Instead, as Brake affirms, "Everyone in a position to save the life of a child has a (*prima facie*) duty to do so."[29] Yet Thomson's case for the permissibility of abor-tion creates other troubles for Brake's case against the causal account. As no few critics have observed, Thomson pictures abortion "as essentially a form of pregnancy termination that involves fetal detachment, rather than as the deliberate termination of the life of the fetus."[30] Uprooting a person-plant, or unplugging yourself from a violinist whose circulatory system has been "plugged into yours, so that your kidneys can be used to extract poison from his blood as well as your own" for the next nine months—Thomson's even more famous example[31]—differs significantly from poisoning, burning, crushing, or dismembering a fetus, which is to say standard methods of abortion.[32] It does not follow from the fact that we would not have a duty to sacrifice nine months of our lives to help save the life of the violinist that we would have a right to poison, burn, crush, or dismember him in order to free ourselves.[33] The example does not even establish that abortion by these methods would be permissible in cases of rape, a conclusion often wrongly conceded by critics distracted by the disanalogy between suddenly finding oneself encumbered by a violinist and finding oneself with child after voluntarily having had sex.[34] Surely, however he got there, we would have to think twice about what the right course of action would be if a famous unconscious violinist were dependent on our bodies as a consequence of actions both not in our control and contrary to our will—but surely again poisoning, burning, crushing, or dismembering him would not be high on the list. Once we try to think some about Thomson's example of the violinist, we really don't know what to think, and the example appears to collapse into irrelevance.

Thomson's example of the person-plant that (who?) has taken root in one's house fares no better. Would it be permissible to poison, burn, crush, or dismember a person-plant, if that is what uprooting it required? I think the answer here should be, to begin with, that we have no idea, since we have no idea what a person-plant is. If it is first and foremost a plant—in other words, in Aristotelian terms, if the kind of soul that animates it is a nutritive soul, such that its life is essentially vegetative—then I suppose we would feel free to do whatever it takes to be rid of it. But if what we have to do with is really a person—well, rather than destroy it (or him or her), why not try to remove it roots and all, so that it might be replanted somewhere else? Persons seem to deserve at least this much consideration. Or, if it is not possible to remove the person roots and all, why not let it (or him or her) live in the house for a while after all? If the only alternative is to poison or crush or burn or dismember him or her, and if what we have to do with really is a person with the same moral standing as the violinist, then none of these courses of action seems like a real alternative at all.

§2. McMAHAN TO THE RESCUE

It might be countered, however, that this objection holds only for methods of abortion that kill the fetus by poisoning, burning, crushing, and dismembering it, and not so-called merely extractive abortions that do not injure or damage the fetus's body in a way that causes death.[35] Jeff McMahan has drawn attention to two such methods of abortion: hysterectomy, when the uterus is removed to terminate the development of a fetus within it (as is performed not infrequently on cats, dogs, and other animals); and hysterotomy, in which a surgical incision is made in the uterus and the fetus is extracted intact. The doctor performing a hysterotomy may first cut the umbilical cord and allow the fetus to die from oxygen deprivation before extracting it, or the doctor may extract the fetus while it is alive and then let it die by withholding life support. To refer to the first type of hysterotomy as an "extractive" abortion is of course misleading, as the fetus dies before extraction; but the important point is that the cause of the fetus's death is not an attack on its body. In this first type of hysterotomy, like the second, the fetus dies for lack of life support, broadly construed. Arguably, merely extractive abortions (to retain this term for abortion by hysterectomy and both types of hysterotomy) closely parallel disconnecting the violinist: merely extractive abortions, it might be claimed, constitute *letting die*, as opposed to killing. It appears to follow that, if letting the violinist die by disconnecting him is permissible, which does seem to be the case, then letting a fetus die by withholding life support, whether before or after extraction, must be likewise permissible. And so Thomson's defense of abortion would suffice for at least these methods of abortion, and Brake's argument would have all the precedent that it needs. (By the way, a more standard method of abortion, namely, the use of mifepristone, formerly known as RU-486, might also be classified as an extractive abortion. Mifepristone blocks the action of the hormone progesterone and changes the uterine lining, such that the fetus becomes detached. The use of the misoprostol then causes the uterus to contract and expel the fetus.)

There is, to say the least, a body of quite complex literature both on the difference between killing and letting die and on the moral significance, if any, of this difference. The standard reference on this question in the medical ethics literature is James Rachels's 1975 article in the *New England Journal of Medicine* on active and passive euthanasia.[36] My own position is that killing and letting die are so-called family resemblance concepts, and that examination of instances of killing and of letting die would reveal in each case not a common core to all such instances, but instead, in Ludwig Wittgenstein's terms, "a complicated network of similarities, overlapping and criss-crossing."[37] In any event, McMahan has recently sought to articulate necessary and jointly sufficient conditions for "letting die" as opposed to "killing," and has applied this account to the question of whether "a merely extractive abortion really involve[s] only allowing the fetus to die rather than killing it."[38] So I focus here on his analysis and argument, which readers should note departs from Rachels's. (To be clear, the point of what follows is to determine whether Brake's argument has the precedent that it needs: her argument for unwilling fathers' "right to choose" parental obligations is baseless unless women have a right to abortion even granting the full moral standing of the fetus.)

McMahan claims that

> Agent does not kill Victim but instead lets Victim die if: (1) there is, independent of anything that Agent might do, some antecedent probability that Victim will die within a certain period; (2) Agent is not responsible for the fact that Victim is thus at risk of death; (3) Victim dies; and (4) Victim could have survived if Agent had provided, or had continued to provide, some form of aid, support, assistance, or protection that it was possible for him to provide—if, in effect, Agent had saved Victim.[39]

McMahan also claims that "to perform a merely extractive abortion—in which the woman does nothing to cause the victim's death other than to remove it from the protective environment through which she has been sustaining its life—is not to kill the fetus but only to let it die." For, according to him, "In removing it, she is simply ceasing to protect it from the consequences of its inability to survive on its own"[40] and instead allowing that "antecedent probability" (condition 1), for which, as such, the woman bears no responsibility (condition 2), to take its natural course to death (condition 3), which was not inevitable but could have been prevented had the woman decided to keep supporting and thus save the fetus (condition 4).

What distinguishes McMahan's account of letting die from Philippa Foot's well-known account is that he denies that, in order for us to have an instance of letting die, the individual in question "must be in the path of a threatening sequence of events that is already in train and is external to his natural state." Instead, he claims that we may also have an instance of letting die "when the only threat the individual faces is a threat latent in his own inherent dependency on aid from the agent."[41] It follows that, on McMahan's account, as he himself points out, parents who fail to feed their baby do not kill it, but let it die.[42] He also says that if we do not replenish the water in a fish tank, but let it evaporate, we do not kill a fish that had been in the tank, but let it die;[43] and again that we do not kill, but let die, if we notice that our boat is pushing toward shore a man who is floating unconscious in the water, but we shove him aside to drown because he is "retarding the progress of [our] cruise."[44] I find all these claims highly counterintuitive. By contrast, Foot claims that such parents, if they can feed the baby but choose not to do so, do not merely let the baby die, but "murder" him or her, which in ordinary language we call killing.[45] (Compare the case of a son who wrongfully extubated his mother. As Richard McCormick has remarked, "He *wrongfully* allowed her to die. Because it was wrong, we easily call it 'killing.'"[46])

McMahan's reason for thinking that Foot is wrong here is that the parents in this case do not create or initiate a threatening sequence of events external to the baby's natural state, but instead withdraw support that they could have provided.[47] As the parents do not create or initiate such a threatening sequence of events, it appears to follow that Foot must say, on her own account, that the parents have *not* killed their baby, such that the use of the term 'murder' is inappropriate here. In other words, inasmuch as Foot holds that it is a necessary condition for us to have an instance of killing that it involve the initiation of a threatening sequence of events external to the baby's natural state, McMahan is right that she must deny that the parents have killed their baby. But why hold—as I do not think that Foot herself does[48]—that the initiation of such a threatening sequence of events is necessary for us to be able to speak of killing? I cannot see why this condition should be considered necessary. Killing may involve the initiation of a threatening sequence of events external to an individual's natural state, but it need not. Surely we can equally well say (and do in ordinary language) that, in some circumstances, another way to kill is to withhold or withdraw life support such that an individual dies, not from some threat "already in train and . . . external to his natural state" that life support had stymied, but precisely because life support has been withheld or withdrawn *when it should not have been*. In other words, another way to *kill* is to let someone wrongfully die.[49]

The qualification "in some circumstances" is important here. Foot gives an example of a case where at least most of us would say that withholding life support and allowing people to die of starvation would *not* constitute killing: namely, should people with money to spare, by choosing to buy a coat rather than give to a charity, thereby allow people in underdeveloped countries to die of starvation. As Foot remarks, "it clearly makes a difference" when we judge whether to speak of killing or letting die whether the "positive duty" to provide care that we bear in a given case is "a strict duty," like that of parents to feed their children, or a rather looser duty, like that to give to charities.[50] It follows that, if we do *not* say that the initiation of a threatening sequence of events external to an individual's natural state is necessary for an instance of killing, it is open to us to say that failing to feed a baby, or to replenish the water in a fish tank, or to bring to the safety of shore a man floating unconscious in the water, each counts as killing rather than merely letting die *inasmuch as*, in each instance, death results from culpable negligence.

As I have already indicated in passing, it should be admitted that there is a sense in which it is right to say that the parents here, the fish's caretaker, and the boater allow the individual in each case to die. What is wrong, however, is to think that these are all cases of letting die *as opposed to* killing. Instead, these are cases of letting die that are also cases of killing; in these instances, as I suggested happens, the concepts cross one another.[51] To put this point in yet another way, all these cases are not cases of *merely* letting die; that is *not* the sense in which it is right to say that the parents, the fish's caretaker, and the boater allow the individual in each case to die. Instead, they are cases of wrongful letting die, and so it makes perfect sense to say in these cases (though with fluctuating levels of passion), You killed that baby! or, You killed that fish! or, You killed that man! And we would rightly reject as sophism the claim that, No, no, I only let the baby, or the fish, or the man die. Disconnecting the violinist, by contrast, would be a case of *merely* letting die, as here the cause of death would be, not as such the withdrawal of life support, but the violinist's preexisting kidney disease, the effects of which had been blocked by his having been plugged into his involuntary benefactor. In other words, here death would be brought about by a threatening sequence of events that is already in train and is external to his natural state.[52]

I think it is also right to say that the doctor performing a hysterotomy, should he or she first cut the umbilical cord, allows the fetus to die from oxygen deprivation; likewise, should the doctor extract the fetus while it is alive, he or she then lets it die by withholding life support. But these likewise are not cases of letting die *as opposed to* killing; instead, in most circumstances, these are cases of letting die that are *also* cases of killing. For here too we would reject as sophism the claim that, No, no, I only let the fetus die. And it would make perfect sense to say, No, you killed it.

It might be countered, however, that the claim that these are cases of letting die that are *also* cases of killing takes for granted that the woman (with the doctor acting as her agent) has a strict duty to the fetus not to let it die, which is to say a duty like that of parents to feed their child, rather than a looser duty like that of the affluent to give to the poor. In other words, it might be countered that a merely extractive abortion should be considered *merely* letting die as opposed to killing. The claim to the contrary must establish that the woman has a strict duty to the fetus not to let it die, such that she would be culpably negligent in the event and that it would make sense, then, to talk of killing (or, if one prefers, wrongful letting die).

In reply, the first point to note is that the case of the violinist, which sent us down this path, is irrelevant to the question at hand. The case of the violinist does not even help us think about a woman's responsibility to a fetus when the woman becomes pregnant by rape. For there is a significant disanalogy between disconnecting the violinist and a merely extractive abortion. When the violinist is disconnected, he dies from a threatening sequence of events that is already in train and is external to his natural state; when the umbilical cord is cut or life support withheld (or mifepristone introduced), the fetus dies, not from a threatening sequence of events already in train and external to its natural state, but precisely from the withdrawal or withholding of life support. So we can agree that letting the violinist die would be morally permissible, without yet gaining any purchase on or insight into what to say about a merely extractive abortion, even if the pregnancy came about by rape (that is, even if it was involuntary in the same way that the violinist's becoming connected was).

A merely extractive abortion is more closely analogous to the exposure, leading to death, of a newborn, taking for granted that a newborn has the full moral standing of a person, as Thomson's argument likewise grants to the fetus. What makes exposure and merely extractive abortion similar is that, in both cases, death is brought about by the withdrawal or withholding of life support, broadly construed. What is different, of course, is that in a merely extractive abortion, before ex utero viability, the fetus can live only within the woman, on whom it makes great demands. After ex utero viability, it is difficult to see all that much difference between letting a fetus die once it has been extracted and exposing a newborn, again taking for granted that they both have the full moral standing of a person. As, normally, exposure surely counts not *merely* as letting die, but also as culpable killing, the conclusion follows that so too would a merely extractive abortion after ex utero viability, and this however the newborn and fetus were conceived, which is to say by consensual sex or by rape. Before ex utero viability, it is more difficult to know what to say about the analogy between a merely extractive abortion and exposure. To repeat, the fetus in utero makes great demands on its mother, but so too, though in different ways, does a newborn. (One important difference, it should be noted, is that care of a newborn, unlike that of a fetus, may be transferred to others.)

If this chapter were about the morality of abortion, at this point, considerations about the facts of human reproduction and family life, and about the proper attitudes toward not only the fetus but human life and death, parenthood, and family relationships—in brief, considerations of virtue and vice—would have to come to the fore.[53] But this chapter is *not* about the morality of abortion. Instead, taking for granted for the sake of argument that the fetus has the full moral standing of a person, the chapter has been focused on the alleged link between the moral permissibility of abortion and the grounds of parental obligations. And so the following analysis can be simpler than a discussion of the morality of abortion would call for. From the point of view of the causal account of parental obligations, *if* it is granted for the sake of argument that a fetus has the full moral standing of a person, it is clear that a pregnant woman would have strict duties to the fetus, before and after ex utero viability, on the condition that she voluntarily acted in such a way that its coming-into-being was a reasonably foreseeable consequence. In other words, the woman would have strict duties if she voluntarily had sex or otherwise acted so that conception became reasonably foreseeable (for example, if she employed IVF). In such a case, it makes sense to think that a merely extractive abortion both before and after ex utero viability would constitute culpable killing rather than merely letting die.

But what about a woman who becomes pregnant by rape? Would she have a strict duty to the fetus (again granting it the full moral standing of a person) not to let it die, such that she would be culpably negligent to remove it from her body before ex utero viability? If we answer no, she does *not* have a strict duty and so would *not* be culpably negligent, then the conclusion follows that she is merely letting the fetus die, rather than also killing it. And it might seem that, at last, Brake's argument from precedent against the causal account has the precedent that it needs: as the woman here does not bear parental responsibility to the fetus despite her role in its coming-into-being, neither can an unwilling father's role ground his responsibility. But this conclusion is mistaken, and the case in question is useless to Brake's argument from precedent against the causal account. The reason why it is not an objection to the causal account that a woman or for that matter a man who is raped and thereby begets a child does not have parental obligations to this child is simple: such a woman or man does not have parental obligations according to the causal account itself as I have presented it. As the causal account claims that parental obligations fall to a person by his or her having *voluntarily* acted in such a way that the coming-into-being of a child was a reasonably foreseeable consequence, the concession that a woman who is raped may rightly have a merely extractive abortion before the fetus is viable ex utero does not call the causal account into question in the least. And no right to a "financial abortion" has been established.

§3. THE REPLY TO (THE REPLY TO) THE RESPONSIBILITY OBJECTION

Readers familiar with the literature on Thomson's argument will know and may even object at this point that there is a final way to defend Brake's argument from precedent. This defense takes issue with my claim that a woman who voluntarily had sex bears responsibility for the fetus who is thereby conceived. To understand this last defense, we need to review briefly another well-known objection to Thomson's argument.

Consider again Thomson's counterexample to the principle that we are morally responsible for *all* the foreseeable consequences of our actions: namely, her story of people-seeds drifting about in the air. Thomson takes for granted here that having sex is *not* the kind of action for which one incurs strict liability, meaning not the kind of action that, because it is inherently risky, makes one responsible for all the reasonably foreseeable consequences of it, even those that we did not intend and took reasonable precautions against. It is true that we do not think of opening one's windows as this kind of action—though, if people-seeds really were drifting around, then opening one's windows would be much more fraught than it now is—but we *do* typically think of sex along these lines. In the United States, for example, strict state child support laws are now the rule.[54]

That having sex is a high-risk action for which one incurs strict liability for the consequences is the heart of the so-called responsibility objection to Thomson's argument. If the responsibility objection is coupled with the claim that a fetus, whether from conception or at some specified time of development, does indeed have the moral standing of a person (so not only for the sake of argument), then we have the beginnings of an argument against elective abortion. If, by contrast, the focus of the objection is not the fetus but the child, then we have not an argument against abortion, but a restatement, in somewhat more bristling terms, of the causal account of parental obligations.[55]

There is, however, a well-known reply to the responsibility objection, and this reply indicates the final way that Brake's argument from precedent might be defended. As Brake concedes, "perhaps mandatory child support should be modelled on strict liability in law, in which someone engaging in a risky activity automatically assumes responsibility for damages, no matter what precaution they [*sic*] have taken." But she replies:

> As Harry Silverstein and David Boonin point out, responsibility for someone's existence is distinct from responsibility for [his or her] being in need. A truck driver who runs down a pedestrian is (causally) responsible for the latter's having urgent medical needs. A pregnant woman is only responsible for the fetus' existence, not its neediness: "[t]here was no option available to [the pregnant woman] on which the fetus would now exist and not be in need of her assistance." As the case of doctors who extend lives shows [an example that is explained shortly below], an agent A's responsibility for B's existence does not imply that B has a right that A do whatever it takes to keep [B] alive (giving up a kidney, for example). This seems to apply to the father too: no more than the mother is he responsible for the *neediness* of the fetus or child, and hence surely he is no more obligated to the child by virtue of his partial responsibility for its existence than the mother is to the fetus.[56]

Whether this defense of "A Defense of Abortion" does in fact suffice, however, is by no means self-evident, despite the reverence with which the argument is often cited. As we have seen in section 2 of this chapter, Thomson's examples do not suffice to establish that it would be justifiable to kill the fetus in order to be free from having to care for it. Instead, if we grant the fetus, as Thomson does, the full moral standing of a person, it seems that, at most, there is an argument to be made that it is morally permissible to let a fetus die by merely extractive abortion in cases of pregnancy by rape before the fetus has become viable ex utero. Now, the reply to the responsibility objection likewise does not establish that it would be justifiable to kill the fetus in order to be free from having to care for it. To speak to the above quotation, I agree that a doctor who has extended a patient's life, and so is in a sense responsible for the patient's existence, is not obligated to do "whatever it takes" to ensure that the patient goes on living. The patient has no such right against the doctor, and the doctor has no such obligation. The heart of the reply to the responsibility objection is that there is a "connection between responsibility and avoidability."[57] In sum, a person who is responsible for another's life—whether by having brought that other into being or by having extended that other's life—bears special responsibility for that other's neediness and so is specially obligated to assist that other only if the person, in the act of giving that other life, could have at the same time avoided the other's being in need, whether that other is a fetus or newborn child who is immediately in need, or a patient who may be in need some time after a doctor's life-giving act.[58] Maybe so—but in any event a doctor in such circumstances may not kill his or her patient. Instead, the doctor is simply not obligated to assume further responsibility for the patient. That is, the doctor may let the patient die.

The reply to the responsibility objection gives us, then, no reason to hold that killing a fetus would be permissible. Moreover, the sense in which a doctor who has extended the life of a patient is responsible for that patient's existence is significantly different from the sense in which a woman who is carrying a fetus is responsible for its existence. The woman, in addition to participating in bringing the fetus into being, is presently sustaining its existence; the doctor acted only to enable the patient to go on living on his or her own. Whereas the question for the doctor, then, is whether he or she is obligated to assume *further* responsibility for the patient—that is, whether he or she is bound to act *again* so that the patient might live longer—the question for the woman is whether it is permissible for her to withdraw her current and ongoing support. As these are quite different questions, answering that the doctor is not obligated to assume further responsibility does not entail, in the terms of the analogy, that the woman is not obligated to carry through with the "course of treatment," so to speak, that she began the fetus on.

The basic problem with the reply to the responsibility objection, however, is that it wrongly denies that the child's neediness was unavoidable. It was unavoidable once the child came into being, but the parents could have avoided bringing the child into being, namely, by not having had sex or otherwise acted to conceive him or her. As McMahan observes, "in order for one to be responsible for an individual's being in a certain state, it does not have to have been possible for the individual to exist without being in that state. All that is necessary is that one could have ensured that the individual would not be in that state"—which one could have done in the present case by not having brought the individual in question into being, for which the mother and father together bear responsibility.[59] And so the reply fails; the responsibility objection stands; and Brake's argument from precedent has, again, no precedent to build on.

A final word is appropriate on Pavlischek's claims regarding the implications of the so-called abortion mentality. If my argument in this chapter is correct, Pavlischek is wrong that Thomson's defense of abortion must lead, *logically*, to the surrender of strict child support laws. Yet it is interesting to find another philosopher—namely, Brake—making just this claim, but with the quite different goal of securing unwilling fathers' "right to choose" whether to take on parental obligations or not. The evidence of Brake's paper suggests that, although "abortion logic" does not in fact undercut the causal account of parental obligations, Pavlischek might not be altogether wrong, in his words again, "that an intimate connection exists between the way we collectively relate to the unborn and the way we relate to children after birth."[60]

NOTE: THE RESPONSIBILITIES OF "DUPED DADS"

This chapter has been concerned with the obligations of so-called unwilling fathers. A neighboring question is what should we think about the obligations, if any, of men who have discovered that they were "duped" into believing that they were the biological fathers of children whom they then contributed to raising. More precisely, do such men retain parental obligations toward these children?

According to many jurisdictions in the United States, so-called duped dads do retain parental obligations, in particular the financial obligations of child support, *unless* they can prove fraud on the part of the woman *and* "demonstrate that upon learning the truth [they] immediately stopped acting as the child's father" by cutting off all ties.[61] Otherwise, courts have reasoned, these men want the benefits of parenthood without the responsibilities.[62]

Take the case of a man who has developed a loving bond with a child whom he then learns is not biologically "his." Would it be morally permissible for him to cut off all ties? Further, is it morally defensible for courts to require men to cut off all ties if they are to be freed of the burden of child support? Yet further, is it right for these men to seek to be freed of this burden to begin with?

Though the details of such a case could make a difference (consider if we were to vary the age of the child and the extent of the father's involvement to date), once a child comes to know and love a man as his or her father, it is difficult to countenance that it could be morally permissible for the man to cut off all ties. The reason is simply that to cut off all ties would be an act of violence toward the child, who after all has not done any wrong and deserves better from someone who loved him or her as a parent. In such a case, it seems that the child is owed love still, though neither because the father begot the child, nor because he voluntarily assumed the obligations of a procreator. Instead, the loving relationship that they have had generates its own reasons why he should go on loving the child as he has, which is to say as a parent. Consider, by way of comparison, whether there is an obligation for close friends to remain friends, or in other words an obligation to stay within the relationship. Unless one party injures the other, there does seem to be such an obligation—but it is an obligation that finds its grounds within the relationship itself, not in some fact outside it.

The conclusion follows that it is likewise not morally defensible for courts to require men to cut off all ties if they are to be freed of the burden of child support. To require a "duped dad" to cut off all ties is to require that he do violence to his child—a child who is not his biologically, as it has been revealed, but was his *effectively* during the years that he believed himself to be the biological father, such that the child retains the right to go on calling him "Dad," and he retains the right, as well as obligation, to go on calling the child his own.

It might well be wondered, however, whether it makes sense to think that a man could be morally justified in cutting off his financial support of a child if the man is not morally justified in cutting off all ties to the child. Some courts have answered: it depends—for example, on whether the mother has since married the biological father of the child, and on whether the child is financially secure. Some judges have also considered the possibility that "a nonbiological father could be granted custody rights," given the history of his relationship with the child, "even if the biological father is charged with paying child support."[63] These solutions seem reasonable. But if a child is not financially secure, it seems no less reasonable that the law should compel a "duped dad" to contribute child support, as in fact many courts have done. What responsibility the public has toward children is a further question here, which I address in the book's closing chapter.

4 Whose Child?

What could be a more private matter, as the United States Supreme Court has intoned more than once over the last several decades, than the decision whether or not to become a parent?[1] Yet, what could be a more public matter than the determination of who counts as a parent and, as such, has the responsibility to do the important and difficult work of raising a child? On the one hand, admittedly, *how* to become a parent is, well, widely known—though it would sadly be quite wrong to take for granted that all persons capable of becoming parents have had adequate sexual education in this regard. But on the other hand, are surrogates— sometimes called surrogate mothers, sometimes merely carriers—parents? This question can be asked whether the surrogacy is "only" gestational (a category that arguably depends for much of its weight on a dubious genetic preformationism: the belief that fetal development is wholly a matter of the unfolding of that fetus's genes), or whether what is at issue is traditional surrogacy—a category that, on second thought, might well strike us as oxymoronic.[2] (In so-called traditional surrogacy, to recall, the mother contributes both genes and gestation, whereas in gestational surrogacy the mother contributes "only" gestation.) Consider next the role that gamete providers, whether sperm or egg, play in conception; should they then be conceived as parents? It might well be countered that, of course, gamete providers are parents—they are *genetic* parents—as likewise gestational surrogates are *gestational* parents, and traditional surrogates are both *genetic* and *gestational* parents. But this terminological maneuver only elides and does not answer the question of who bears parental responsibilities to the child born. A surrogate or provider might well claim that she or he is not *really* the parent of a child whom she or he helped bring into being. What this claim means, translated from the vernacular, is that she or he does not have parental responsibilities with respect to this child; someone else is *really* the parent in this sense, meaning the responsibilities of parenting fall elsewhere.

The present chapter engages the host of controversies that have sprung up since the development of IVF—what one author calls Pandora's baby.[3] As I indicated in my introduction and in chapter 2, a common charge against the causal account is that it is useless in the assignment of parental responsibility in the age of new reproductive technologies, given how many parties may play crucial, "but-for" roles in the coming-into-being of a child. (A person plays a "but-for" role if it is the case that, but for or without him or her, this or that effect would not have come to pass.) In the normal case of procreation, namely, sex between a woman and a man, the critic of the causal account would be hard pressed to make a plausible case that the couple in question should *not* be considered the proximate cause of the child's coming-into-being, or that considering the couple the proximate cause is somehow arbitrary or merely "conventional" in any significant sense. In cases involving reproductive technologies, there is significantly less certainty in this regard. (By the way, I classify surrogacy as a reproductive technology inasmuch as, nowadays, even so-called traditional surrogates typically become pregnant by what we might call non-natural means.[4])

§1. PANDORA'S BABIES

Consider, by way of example, whether a gestational surrogate should be accounted as a parent, in particular a mother to the child whom she gestates and bears. Notably, gestational surrogates are themselves more than likely to deny that they bear parental responsibilities to the children they help bring into being. In a *New York Times Magazine* article that drew much attention, one gestational surrogate was quoted casting herself as only "the 'foster mother' to the baby until it is born" and referring to herself by the nickname "the Easy-Bake oven," with the implication that her only contribution to a pregnancy is to "cook" ingredients prepared by others.[5] This language is consistent with that of the surrogacy industry, the promoters of which sometimes describe surrogates' labor in impersonal terms and the surrogates themselves "as inanimate objects: mere 'hatcheries,' 'plumbing,' or 'rented property,'" with accordingly no intelligible claims to the resulting products.[6] A similar position is found as well in the philosophical literature: according to one author, the gestational surrogate is no more than "a foster mother or . . . a wet nurse who cares for a child when the natural mother cannot or does not do so."[7]

Gestational surrogates have, of course, a financial interest in speaking this way: a sure way for a would-be surrogate *not* to be employed would be for her to insist in her application that she would be as much a mother of the child-to-be carried and born as, let us call her, the genetic mother would be. Arguably, gestational surrogates might also have a psychological interest in speaking this way. As Elizabeth Anderson has observed, "Many social expectations and considerations surround women's gestational labor, marking it off as an occasion for the parents to prepare themselves to welcome a new life into their family" and seeking "to encourage parental love for the child." Anderson cites the common example that "obstetricians use ultrasound not simply for diagnostic purposes but also to encourage maternal bonding with the fetus." By contrast, the commercial surrogate, who after all is paid not only to carry and birth but to relinquish the child, must work against "a norm of parenthood," namely, "that during pregnancy one create a loving attachment to one's child," in favor instead of "a norm of commercial production," namely, "that the producer shall not form any special emotional ties to her product" lest she be unwilling or even in some way unable to part with it.[8] It makes sense to think that one way to make this form of "emotional labor" a little easier would be to deny that one is *really* a parent at all.

Finally, gestational surrogates may speak this way of themselves, and be spoken of this way by others, for what might be called historical reasons. The long history of sexism found powerful expression in Aristotle's biological writings, in particular his theory of generation. According to Aristotle, as Susan Okin has put it, "It is the male who performs the active role [in providing the form or soul via his semen], whereas the female merely acts as a passive receptacle for the new life," which takes nutrients from her, but is in its essential being independent from her.[9] The important point for present purposes is that gestation is conceived here as playing a developmental role in the strictest sense: gestation on this account is "literally the unfolding or unrolling of something that is already present and in some way preformed" (hence the term preformationism).[10] On this account, a woman's contribution is merely to provide a place and some stuff—food and other matter—for this process to take place. Of course, we no longer hold Aristotle's biology, or believe, with later scientists, that the adult organism is contained in miniature in either the sperm or egg. As Richard Lewontin has noted, however, much "modern developmental biology is framed . . . in terms of genes and cell organelles, while environment plays only the role of a background factor." And so much modern developmental biology remains basically preformationist, with a difference "only of . . . mechanical details" from earlier theories.[11] Such genetic preformationism, which has gained popular currency, underwrites the conception of gestational surrogacy as analogous to foster care, or, though the image is even more demeaning, baby-sitting for someone else's admittedly quite demanding child. On this account, the gestational surrogate is Aristotle's mere receptacle.[12]

Epigenetic theories that stress the parallel developmental role of gene and environment, in particular the prenatal environment, have put genetic preformationism on the defensive.[13] It looks to be a moot question, however, just how "essential" the contribution of the prenatal environment is to a child's biological constitution and identity. In the philosophical literature, an argument is made that, though "both genetic and gestational parents play a role in creating the child . . ., it is only the genetic parents who play an essential role," as one and the same individual could have had a different gestational mother, but could not have developed from a different sperm and egg, which is to say from different genetic material.[14] Maybe so, but epigenetic, in utero modification of gene function means this argument cannot be considered self-evident, and in any event, as Tim Bayne and Avery Kolers have remarked, when "we ask about the *real* creators of jointly produced objects, or objects the different parts of which are contributed by different partial-creators, it seems arbitrary to insist that the only *real* creators are those who supply the essential features of the thing in question," which is to say those parts that cannot be replaced without changing the thing's identity. Yes, supplying irreplaceable parts does appear *sufficient* to be counted as a creator; but what reason is there to hold that supplying irreplaceable parts is also *necessary* to be so counted?[15] Why should it not suffice to supply replaceable but still literally vital parts—let us say for simplicity's sake, after Aristotle, matter? This argument does not, then, establish that only the genetic parents count as the "real" parents of a child. Advocates of the claim that only gestational parents count as real parents point out, by contrast, that "the [fetus] is *physically contained* within" the woman who gestates it, "*physiologically integrated*" with her, and "*materially derived*" from her body. The fetus may then be considered "part of the woman's body," and what more needs to be established in order to show that it is properly hers?[16] The problem with this argument is that it does not follow from the fact—if we even want to grant that it is a fact, which is certainly questionable—that a fetus is "part of the woman's body" that she is then its real parent to the exclusion of the persons from whom the fetus is generically derived. To quote Bayne and Kolers again, "there is little prima facie reason" to regard material derivation as having priority over genetic derivation—though they claim that this statement also holds vice versa. According to Bayne and Kolers, "Arguments from derivation support [what they call] sufficiency gestationalism"—that is, that gestating a child suffices to count as his or her parent—"but [these arguments] also support [what they call] sufficiency geneticism"—that is, that passing down one's genes to a child suffices to make one his or her parent.[17]

Some people would agree intuitively that gestating a child suffices to make one a parent in the full sense, with parental responsibilities and rights;[18] others, however, would disagree, these others including, most notably, gestational surrogates. They are certainly vital causes in the coming-into-being of a child; but what are we to say if they insist that they are, nonetheless, not *really* parents to the children whom they help produce? Intuitions are no longer of any use, and arguably even the concept of 'parent' is no longer useful here. It applies easily enough when only one man and one woman play the biological roles—this case, we might say, is the concept's natural home—but seems to lose its hold in cases involving new reproductive technologies with multiple parties playing "but-for" roles. These cases suggest that the concept 'parent' has what the legal theorist H.L.A. Hart called "a fringe of vagueness or 'open texture,'" with "a core of certainty and a penumbra of doubt," which he claimed all general terms have.[19] We can *choose* to call, for example, a gestational surrogate or a gamete provider a parent (somewhat more authoritatively, a legislature could so choose); but there is no use pretending that we could not have chosen otherwise—as if the concept gave us no choice by laying down in advance the lines of our thought.

In order to move beyond the clash of intuitions, what we need is a *theory* of how parental obligations are acquired—which of course is just what the causal account of parental obligations, elaborated in chapter 2 and defended in chapter 3, is. According to the formulation of the causal account that I have presented, women and men incur parental obligations by voluntarily acting in such a way that the coming-into-being of a child was a reasonably foreseeable consequence in the normal course of events. So, according to this formulation, it is not the case that all parties who play crucial, "but-for" roles in the coming-into-being of a child incur parental obligations. We can eliminate, for example, pro-natalist friends, pushy would-be grandparents, and purveyors of fine bottles of wine from the list of candidates for parental obligations. Extolling the joys of children, clamoring for grandchildren, and contributing to the mood for less than fully careful romance do not amount to effecting the coming-into-being of a child. More precisely, as much as pro-natalist friends and pushy would-be grandparents might wish to the contrary, none of these actions has the coming-into-being of a child as a reasonably foreseeable consequence in the normal course of events. Instead, extolling children and clamoring for grandchildren provide considerations in view of which the responsible agents may act. Providing a fine bottle of wine does not make agents act carelessly, but may figure in careless action if the responsible agents drink the wine and, under its influence, give themselves over to the moment.

It also follows according to this formulation, however, that so-called intended or sponsoring parents (the terminology varies), gamete providers, and both traditional and gestational surrogates *all* incur parental obligations to children. Moreover, so too do clinicians, technicians, and the like—which might well seem absurd. Against these claims, it might be countered that gamete providers and surrogates, and all the more intended or sponsoring parents, play in some sense "greater" roles in the coming-into-being of a child than clinicians and technicians do. This certainly seems right at first sight, but I agree with David Archard that the response in turn is that "it is a mistake to conflate the empirical or metaphysical question of the degree of causal influence (what or who played the most significant role in bringing X about) with the normative question of the degree of moral or legal responsibility for X."[20] And it might be claimed further that defenders of the causal account who see some causes (say, intended parents or gamete providers or surrogates) as "more primary" than others (say, clinicians and technicians and the like) "court the risk of simply reading off the degree of individuals' moral or legal responsibility for the child's care from the magnitude or salience of [these individuals'] causal contribution to [the child's] existence."[21] Such defenders so also court the charge that the problem of why some ways of causing a child's existence bring parental obligations, whereas others do not, has not been solved, but simply waved away by appeal to pre-reflective prejudices.[22]

My aim in what follows is to lend credibility to the claim that intended or sponsoring parents, gamete providers, surrogates, and clinicians, technicians, and the like *all* incur *procreative costs* by doing what they do. The language of the "costs of procreation" and "procreative costs," introduced in chapter 2, is helpful here because it allows us to bypass endless debates about whether surrogates, gamete providers, and clinicians and technicians can really, meaningfully be called parents and so considered candidates for parental obligations. As I noted in chapter 2, speaking in terms of the costs of procreation and procreative costs has the advantage of focusing attention on the sum of obligations one incurs by bringing a child into being—whether we would want to call the parties to this act parents or not (that is, whether the language of *parental* obligations seems to fit or not). The concept of 'procreator' has no doubt an "open texture" just as the concept of 'parent' does, but little hangs on whether we find it natural or not to call gestational surrogates and gamete providers, and clinicians and technicians, "procreators." Instead, what matters is if these persons play relevant causal roles in a child's coming-into-being—which I go on now to examine more closely.

§2. YOU ARE THE (WO)MAN!

I begin with gamete donation, since it is often cited as a challenge to the causal account. The use of the term 'donation' for what gamete providers do has several effects. First, it suggests that providing sperm and eggs is an altruistic deed, which of course for some persons it may well be, though for others it may be wholly mercenary.[23] Second, it sidesteps the question of whether it is appropriate to conceive of gametes as property and so to pay providers not merely for services rendered, but for the gametes themselves.[24] Currently, the money that passes hands typically goes under the name of compensation, though the great variation in sums, for eggs in particular, makes this language hard to take seriously.[25] Third, the use of the term 'donation' also suggests that providers incur no costs in providing gametes—in other words, that the transaction is only and all about giving, essentially the same as giving blood, which once it is done (it is typically thought) is simply done, responsibility for the use of the product falling then to others. On this understanding, gamete providers incur no procreative costs; in other words, they are absolved altogether of any share of parental responsibilities or obligations.

Much of the philosophical literature on gamete donation is focused on the question of under what circumstances it is permissible for a provider to alienate or, perhaps more charitably, transfer responsibility for his or her gametes and whatever children result from these gametes. David Benatar argues that "gamete donation is almost always morally deficient," as responsibilities for rearing children are weighty, and at present the majority of gamete providers transfer these responsibilities "without even knowing the identity, let alone any details, of those who will rear their genetic children," thereby showing a "lack of seriousness" about these responsibilities.[26] By contrast, some philosophers concerned with the grounds of parental obligations simply take for granted that gamete donation is cost free to the provider. For example, in opposition to the causal account, Brake exclaims, "think of sperm donors!"[27] Others have concurred but given reasons for this position. Tim Bayne has proposed that we should regard the gamete provider not "as transferring his or her *parental* claims over any offspring resulting from [the] gametes," but instead "as transferring [his or her] *property* claims over the gametes" and therewith only "potential parental responsibilities," which, once actualized with the coming-into-being of a child, fall to the persons who used the gametes to this end.[28] Bayne accordingly (and colorfully) likens the gamete provider to a man who donates a testicle to another man (called, in the literature, a "gonadal transplant," which is possible as well for ovarian tissue, though at present both these procedures remain in development). If this other man then takes part in begetting a child, Bayne claims that "intuitively" it is this man, rather than the provider, who ought to be held responsible for the offspring.[29] The same holds, Bayne thinks, for a person who uses donated gametes: as the gametes come to belong to him or her, so too should responsibility for any child whom they are used to produce. The upshot is that gamete donation is cost free to the provider; all procreative costs fall to others. Yet, as Giuliana Fuscaldo has observed, Bayne's account is vulnerable to the objection that it excludes "too much from the realm of consequences for which we can be held accountable."[30] Because it is clearly foreseeable that gamete donation will likely result in the birth of a child, it is "problematic to claim that gamete donors are not morally accountable for consequences that follow from their donation" on the grounds simply that they transferred possession and control of these gametes to others.[31]

From the point of view of the causal account, which can be represented here by quoting James Nelson's succinct summary, the decisive consideration is that (premise 1) gamete donation "is an act highly proximate to conception, and, in concert with the other parent's action, is jointly sufficient for it."[32] Moreover (premise 2), "Our practice is generally to take proximity and sufficiency pretty seriously" in the assignment of moral responsibility for an event. For "a pair of coordinated actions which were proximate to and jointly sufficient for an event, and were not the result of forcing or fraudulent action on the part of others, would be hard not to see as *the* cause of the event in question,"[33] and one bears moral responsibility for the consequences that, in the normal course of events, come about from one's voluntary actions. As (premise 3) gamete providers (and traditional surrogates) voluntarily make available their gametes, the conclusion follows that gamete providers (and traditional surrogates) are morally responsible for children conceived and born from their gametes.

In support of this conclusion, given the critical role of genetics in a person's development and constitution, it seems indisputable that a gamete provider has much to answer for in presuming to help bring a child into being. Consider an example. Jeff McMahan poses the case of a sperm donor who, on donating his sperm, "signs an agreement that both guarantees him anonymity and absolves him of all responsibility for any child who might be conceived using his sperm."[34] Such an agreement is surely problematic. What if the child has a rare disease that the provider can help cure, say by donating bone marrow? Surely the provider, qua procreator, has a special reason to help the child, beyond any reasons that a general duty of beneficence might yield.[35] And what if the provider recklessly or even knowingly fails to disclose the likelihood of his passing down a debilitating genetic condition?[36] Surely he should bear responsibility for the evil that he wreaks.

Yet we need to consider a basic objection. Cynthia Cohen has claimed that "[i]t is incorrect . . . to assert that sperm donors," and presumably egg donors as well, "cause the birth of their biological children."[37] Her reasoning is that, unlike "the man who impregnates a woman by means of sexual intercourse," whose act of directly injecting sperm into the woman's uterus is sufficient to the end of causing the coming-into-being of a child, the sperm donor merely "provides [sperm] to others who must carry out many additional tasks before the sperm reaches the uterus—if it does."[38] This objection may be put more strongly in the terminology of action theory. Consider the claim that, inasmuch as an action is not just a bodily movement but instead is identical with "the causing of each and every consequence to which the doer's agency in doing it extends," one bears moral responsibility for the consequences that come about from one's voluntary actions *just because these consequences are one's actions.*[39] This claim requires, however, at least two qualifications. First, one's agency is cut short, so to speak, by the intervention of other agents. Second, one's agency does not extend to abnormal events.[40] For a relevant example, consider this quite colorful case, which has the extra merit of allegedly having come to pass: "A man tells a woman with whom he is having an affair that he does not want to have children. Throughout the course of the relationship they engage only in oral sex, [but] during one occasion . . . she, unbeknownst to him, retains his sperm" and subsequently impregnates herself with it.[41] It seems reasonable to hold that, as conception is not a reasonably foreseeable consequence of oral sex in the normal course of events, and as the man's action was not sufficient to the end of causing the coming-into-being of a child but had this consequence only as a result of the woman's intervening actions, he cannot be considered a proximate cause of the child's coming-into-being and so is not morally responsible for the child (though I think it is imaginable that he might feel he has some reason to take an interest in the child).[42] Cohen's point about sperm donors (and egg donors as well) can be put in similar terms: as the coming-into-being of a child occurs, if it does at all, only with the intervention of other agents (including clinicians, technicians, and the like), providers cannot rightly be considered proximate causes and so cannot rightly be assigned moral responsibility for any resulting children. For providers' agency is "cut short" by the intervention of other agents.

In response, it should be noted to begin with that an implication of Cohen's objection is that male *partners* (husbands, significant others, and the like) who provide sperm for use in artificial insemination should likewise not be considered proximate causes of the birth of their biological children, since in these cases as well (to quote Cohen) the man merely "provides [sperm] to others who must carry out many additional tasks before the sperm reaches the uterus—if it does." On this logic, the partner would be within his rights to disclaim obligations to the child, which seems counterintuitive. Perhaps it could be claimed that the partner incurs obligations to his child because, in participating in artificial insemination, he somehow promises the woman to parent the child with her; but on this account the man would have obligations to the child only indirectly, because of his obligations to the woman, who it follows could free the man of his obligations to the child by releasing him from his promise. This implication, too, seems counterintuitive. Yes, the man has caused the woman to be with child; but he has also caused the child, to whom he is then likewise responsible. What right does the woman have to waive the man's responsibilities on behalf of the child? Finally, perhaps it could be claimed that the partner incurs obligations to the child because, after all, the partner participates in artificial insemination with the aim of bringing a child into being. So too, however, does a donor, and so this last claim gives us no means to distinguish the cases in question.

Where Cohen goes wrong can be appreciated by another, more traditional example. While the Israelites were attacking the Ammonites, David, the Israelites' king, "was sitting in Jerusalem" with all too much time on his hands.[43] There he saw, from the roof of his palace, a beautiful woman bathing, Bathsheba the wife of Uriah, a warrior in David's army. David sent for her and had sex with her, and she became pregnant. David then called Uriah back from the front and sought to persuade him to sleep with his wife. But Uriah refused—"The ark and Israel and Judah are sitting in huts . . ., and shall I then come to my house to eat and to drink and to lie with my wife?"[44]—so David sent him back to the front, but with a letter for the commander Joab. In this letter David had written, "Put Uriah in the face of the fiercest battling and draw back, so that he will be struck down and die."[45] Joab complied with the king's command, and Uriah was killed by the Ammonites. Now, does not responsibility for his death lie also with Joab and all the more with David, who orchestrated his death and as such was its principal agent? So the prophet Nathan, telling David a story of a rich man who stole from a poor man his prized ewe, led David to see:

> And David's anger flared hot against the [rich] man, and he said to Nathan, "As the Lord lives, doomed is the man who has done this! And the poor man's ewe he shall pay back fourfold, in as much as he has done this thing, and because he has no pity!" And Nathan said to David, "You are the man!"[46]

I do not present this example as an analogy. After all, whereas David orchestrated Uriah's death and so bore ultimate responsibility for it (David desired it, Joab did so only for David), the gamete provider does not orchestrate the coming-into-being of a child—but he or she does wittingly and voluntarily play a critical part to this end. (Unlike Joab, the provider desires the end him or herself, though he or she does not carry it out as Joab does.) The point, then, is that other agents (including clinicians, technicians, and the like) do not "cut short" providers' agency. Instead, to the contrary, these other agents *extend* providers' agency—that is, work to bring it about that what providers deliberately contributed toward comes to pass. Cohen's objection does not, then, counter Nelson's claim that the making available of one's gametes, by a partner or a donor alike, is an action "highly proximate" to conception.

Surrogacy presents similar considerations. Whether they are traditional or gestational, surrogates act, of course, at the behest of the intended or sponsoring parents. Thinking along these lines, Seana Shiffrin claims that intended or "sponsoring parents' primary role in initiating creation with the intent to care for the child" gives courts reason to consider these parents the presumptive holders of custody rights in cases of conflict.[47] That commercial surrogates "earlier . . . viewed the creation as a financial transaction, not a responsibility-generating event," Shiffrin reasons, "provides grounds for presuming"—though defeasibly—"that the sponsoring parents have had a stronger and less wavering commitment to the child's best interests" and so might best be entrusted with these interests.[48] Shiffrin also sees advantages to considering the intended parents the preferred holders of a duty of support. A reason to rest primary duties of support with intended parents is to ensure that they cannot legally reject a child at birth should he or she disappoint expectations.[49] A reason *not* to rest primary duties of support with surrogates is that they normally would not be prepared to assume these duties, since they had not intended or expected to assume these duties in acting as surrogates.

That there are presumptive reasons for a court to assign parental rights and responsibilities to intended parents is not to say, however, that surrogacy should be considered "cost free." As I have noted already, whether a gestational surrogate figures as a necessary condition for the coming-into-being of a particular child—in other words, whether the very same child could, in principle, have come into being via a different gestational surrogate—is a matter of dispute that seems unlikely to be resolved. Yet a surrogate, just by virtue of gestating a child and so apart from whether she is also the child's genetic parent, is profoundly bound up in the child's coming-into-being. What the surrogate consumes, how she takes care of herself, and what she experiences while carrying the child all bear on him or her.[50] Not only does whether the child is born lie in the surrogate's hands; there is much that she can do to affect the conditions of the child's life, for good and for ill. Against this background, it is reasonable to think that, should a child's intended parents die, disappear, or be found incompetent, a court might, in case of need, assign parental obligations to the surrogate. As precedent for such a decision, courts have already recognized both traditional and gestational surrogates as full, legal parents when the women decided against relinquishing the children whom they bore.[51]

Finally, imagine a child who asks clinicians et al. why he or she exists. They might well reply by pointing the child to his or her intended parents, gamete providers, or surrogate. Such a reply makes good sense inasmuch as clinicians et al. work at the behest of intended parents, work to bring it about that what providers contributed toward comes to pass, and work with surrogates in service of the intended parents' end—yet there is also no denying that what clinicians et al. do is to cause, in concert with these other agents, the coming-into-being of a child. Accordingly, clinicians et al. have to answer for, not only the quality of the work they do,[52] but having agreed to work for the intended parents to begin with. Moreover, Dr. Frankenstein is a salutary reminder that, should for example human reproductive cloning become feasible, clinicians et al. might in fact be the principal candidates for the responsibilities of rearing the resulting child. For there might be no one else who did the deed. Whether it would be in the child's best interests to live with such parents could well be doubted, but I do not think it can be doubted that the clinicians et al. in such a case would have much to answer for. Frankenstein abjectly failed to take responsibility for his creation—as I noted in this book's introduction, egregiously, it was not until some nine months *after* the animation of the creature that Frankenstein "[f]or the first time . . . felt what the duties of a creator towards his creature were"[53]—but there is no question that he had such duties.

§3. THE TRANSFER PRINCIPLE, TAKE TWO

At the end of my chapter 1, I discussed reasons to be wary of—though not to reject altogether—the so-called *"transfer principle*, according to which it is permissible to alienate one's parental responsibilities (over neonates) to another individual (or institution) as long as one has good reason to think that [the individual or institution] will carry out those responsibilities adequately," without need for further justification, such as that one is mentally or financially incapable of meeting the responsibilities oneself.[54] I also noted that at the bottom of the transfer principle is the supposition that what procreators owe a child is to see to it that he or she is cared for, not necessarily to care for the child themselves.[55] I stand by the arguments of chapters 1 and 2 that procreation brings with it prima facie parental obligations that it would be wrong to alienate or transfer simply at will, which is to say without good reason. It might seem to follow from these arguments that, as Lisa Cahill has claimed, separation of biological and social parenthood is justified only "when the motivating factor is the best interests of the child, and when the circumstances requiring the separation are preexisting and now beyond human control."[56] In other words, more concretely, it might seem to follow that, while relinquishing a child for adoption can be justified under some circumstances, gamete donation and surrogacy can rarely if ever be justified inasmuch as, in these practices, the separation of biological and social parenthood is planned in advance of the conception of the child.

This conclusion may well be right. In other words, I do not reject it out of hand, as it is certainly not *inconsistent* with my arguments to this point. Yet I also think that it is too hastily drawn.

Let it be conceded, as I have argued, that procreation brings with it prima facie parental obligations that it would be wrong to alienate or transfer simply at will, which is to say without good reason. Against this background, the clear question to ask with respect to gamete donation and surrogacy is whether helping would-be parents have a child could count as a sufficiently "good reason." After all, helping competent, loving would-be parents have a child not only would bring these parents satisfaction; it would also, one would hope, bring a highly valuable relationship into the world, namely, that between the parents and the child. And of course it would give a child life. The rub here is that, if, as I have claimed, life is a mixed benefit, compromised by risks and inevitable burdens, doing good by would-be parents is not doing good enough. Procreators bear responsibilities to the child-to-be that also have to be taken into account.

One way to approach the question of whether helping would-be parents have a child could count as a sufficiently "good reason" to justify the separation of biological and social parenthood is to emphasize the fact that parental obligations or duties are prima facie, which is to say obligations or duties that obtain not absolutely, but on the condition that there are not overriding considerations. The next point to note is that having a child is a great good for persons who yearn for children and that a loving parent-child relationship is a great good to bring to the world. (As for whether would-be parents who turn to gamete donation or surrogacy *should* instead adopt because there are already many children in need of loving homes, it is not always noted that this objection must apply as well to couples who do not have any trouble conceiving.[57]) So perhaps it could be claimed, as Michael Austin has done, that the interests of would-be parents, as well as the interests of providers or surrogates to help would-be parents, present countervailing considerations sufficient to override providers' and surrogates' obligations to the children so born.[58]

This approach needs, however, critical consideration. To begin with, it appears to play a bit fast and loose with the concept of a prima facie duty. As W.D. Ross introduced it, a prima facie duty is binding unless there is another, conflicting duty that, all things considered, ought to take priority as what he terms our *actual* duty in the circumstances. So, for example, if one makes a promise, one is obligated to keep that promise unless it conflicts with some other duty that one judges, in the circumstances, "more incumbent" on one, such as preventing serious harm to others.[59] Giving up a child for adoption may be justified in these terms. When a parent is unprepared or incompetent for the duties of parenting, the duty of beneficence, or for that matter the duty of nonmaleficence, may warrant and even obligate the parent to part with his or her child. It seems difficult, however, to justify current practices of gamete donation and surrogacy in similar terms. For, what conflicting duty ought to take priority over the procreators' duties to the children whom they help bring into being? Perhaps gamete providers and surrogates could point to the duty of beneficence—after all, gamete donation and surrogacy redound to the good of would-be parents, who may be yearning for a child and wary of adoption[60]—but this suggestion might be challenged given that currently, for many providers and surrogates, it is money rather than beneficence that is the decisive motivating factor (though altruism may figure as well).

However these considerations shake out, a more promising approach is to ask whether or not there is or could be so-called *proportionate reason* in favor of these new ways of making babies. The criteria of proportionate reason received much attention from twentieth-century Roman Catholic moral theologians concerned with the proper understanding of the principle of double effect. Richard McCormick was an important figure in this debate, and his formulation of the criteria is both representative and oft-cited. (By the way, what one makes of the principle of double effect is irrelevant here; I am interested in the criteria of proportionate reason, not the validity of double-effect reasoning.[61])

According to McCormick:

> *Proportionate reason means three things*: (a) a value at least equal to that sacrificed is at stake; (b) there is no less harmful way of protecting the value here and now; (c) the manner of its protection here and now will not undermine it in the long term.[62]

McCormick also states the criteria negatively:

> An action is disproportionate in any of the following instances: [a] if a lesser value is preferred to a more important one; [b] if evil is unnecessarily caused in the protection of a greater good; [c] if, in the circumstances, the manner of protecting the good will undermine it in the long run.[63]

Admittedly, the assessment of gamete donation and surrogacy in light of these criteria is likely to be as controversial as the assessment of whether or not the interests of would-be parents suffice to override procreators' prima facie obligations. These criteria offer the advantage, however, of focusing the debate. To begin with, that helping others have a child is a great good appears difficult to deny; whether (a) its value is "at least equal" to the value to be "sacrificed," namely, the value of a biologically based parent-child relationship, is open to dispute. We have to consider, too, whether traditional and gestational surrogacy should be evaluated differently in this regard. That is, is more sacrificed when a genetic tie is lost, or just as much when "only" a gestational tie is at stake?

Whether (b) there is "no less harmful way" for would-be parents to have a child than through current practices of gamete donation or surrogacy is likewise open to dispute. Adoption, of course, is often presented as a better alternative, but it has been countered that adoption, in any event as currently practiced in the United States, "does not unproblematically serve the interests of all parties in the adoption triangle as is commonly supposed."[64] Some would-be parents, as well and for whatever reason, want a genetic tie with the child they are to raise, a wish that, however it is assessed (and certainly it should not be trivialized), adoption normally cannot satisfy.

Finally, as to (c) whether the practices of gamete donation and surrogacy threaten to undermine the good that they seek to serve—the good of the parent-child relationship, or more simply family—there are consequentialist arguments in the literature making just this case. For example, Daniel Callahan claims that the "nullification of the moral obligations that ought to go with biological fatherhood . . . contribute[s] to the further infantilization of males, a phenomenon already well-advanced in our society, and itself a long-standing source of harm for women." Accordingly, "Women who use males in this way [that is, as anonymous sperm providers] cannot fail to do harm both to women and parenthood."[65] One of Elizabeth Anderson's arguments against commercial surrogacy has a similar cast: "To recognize the legitimacy of commercial surrogate contracts," she claims, "would undermine the integrity of families by giving public sanction to a practice which expresses contempt for the moral and emotional ties which bind a mother to her children."[66] Yet these worries appear vulnerable to rejection as exaggerated. Skeptics might well ask whether it is really the case that the practices of sperm donation and commercial surrogacy risk unleashing such systemic consequences.[67] Instead, it might be claimed that, despite occasional highly publicized controversies (for example, when a surrogate changes her mind), assessment of the consequences points, on the whole, in favor of these practices given the great goods that they bring to would-be parents.

Reflection on these considerations leads, I think, to several conclusions. The first, which is hardly novel, is that gamete donation and surrogacy must be assessed independently of one another. Though they can be characterized in ways that emphasize similarities—traditional surrogacy can even be described as gamete donation in utero[68]—there is reason to wonder whether the differences between the practices might make a moral difference, in particular with respect to the first and second criteria of proportionate reason that (a) a lesser value is not preferred to a greater one, and that (b) evil is not to be unnecessarily caused. (I return to this point.)

The second conclusion pertains to gamete donation. This is that there appear to be *circumstances* in which gamete providers might help bring a child into being, but then legitimately leave most procreative costs to others while keeping faith with the child-to-be-born. In other words, I think there is reason to affirm, with respect to gamete donation, a qualified version of the so-called transfer principle.

On my reckoning, five necessary and jointly sufficient conditions must be met:

1. The gamete provider has good reason to believe that the other, intended parent or parents would fulfill their obligations;[69]
2. The provider agrees to make available, promptly and fully, all relevant medical information as it is discovered;
3. The provider agrees to be him or herself available and, within reason, willing to assume responsibility should the child have a special medical need that the provider either is specially placed to help with or negligently caused (recall McMahan's example of the gamete provider whose offspring suffers from a rare disease that the provider is specially placed to help cure);
4. The provider agrees to have his or her identity revealed when the child comes of age; and
5. The provider agrees to meet with the child at that point, *should* the child seek to meet; to discuss with the child his or her origins; and to develop with the child an appropriate relationship, *if* that is what the child wants and needs.

My reason for thinking that gamete donation *could be* warranted under these circumstances is drawn from what little data we have about the experiences and thinking of persons conceived through it. According to a recent study published by the politically conservative Institute for American Values, a majority of these persons experience struggles with identity comparable to those of many adopted persons (as documented in chapter 1). The study found that, "on average, young adults conceived through sperm donation are hurting more, are more confused, and feel more isolated from their families" than peers raised by biological parents.[70] In particular, donor offspring are "about 1.5 times more likely . . . to report mental health problems" and "more than twice as likely . . . to report substance abuse problems."[71] Further, approximately two-thirds support the donor offspring's right to know the identity of his or her father and to form a relationship with him, which in most countries is not the rule.[72] The study *also* found, however, that 61 percent of donor offspring "say they favor the practice of donor conception (compared to 39 percent of adopted children and 38 percent raised by their biological parents)" and, even more remarkably, that a full 20 percent of donor offspring reported that they had themselves already donated sperm or eggs or served as a surrogate, "compared to 0 percent of the adopted adults [surveyed] and just 1 percent of those raised by their biological parents."[73]

I take these last findings to suggest that, from the perspective of a good number of donor offspring (who have a claim to be taken seriously in this matter), the goods realized by gamete donation generally offset the losses. In other words, in terms of criterion (a) of proportionate reason, "a value at least equal to that sacrificed is at stake." At the same time, it cannot be overlooked that a good number of donor offspring have suffered from current practices of gamete donation. We also have reason, then, to advocate change—as indicated in my five conditions—lest evil be unnecessarily caused, in violation of criterion (b). Finally, so long as providers retain some responsibilities—that is, so long as procreation is not "cost free"—I think that worries, like Callahan's, about the degradation of parenthood can be forestalled, thus satisfying criterion (c), that the manner of realizing the good in question (here a parent-child relationship) not undermine it in the long term.

As for putting my five conditions into practice, we need to ask with respect to condition 1: what would constitute "good reason" to believe that the other, intended parent or parents would fulfill their obligations? Knowing the prospective parents personally might well suffice, as when a provider is, say, a close friend or a cousin (though such an arrangement no doubt presents challenges of its own); but how much assurance, and of what kind, would be required from an intermediary agency or institution? In other words, who would do the vetting, and with what criteria? Further, who would determine, and again with what criteria, whether providers understood, took seriously, and were adequately prepared for the responsibilities, though limited, that they were about to assume? Condition 2 (prompt and ongoing disclosure of relevant medical information) raises difficult questions of privacy and confidentiality. Morally, the provider might be obligated to share all relevant medical information as it is discovered, but whether he or she could be legally compelled to do so is perhaps doubtful. Condition 3 (the provider agrees to assume responsibility should the child have a special medical need) prompts the question: how much responsibility? Further, here again morality and the law appear to part ways. Morally, the gamete provider in McMahan's example might have an obligation to donate bone marrow, but it is difficult, as well as disturbing, to imagine a legal system seeking to enforce such an obligation. Finally, condition 5 (the provider agrees to meet with the child and to develop an appropriate relationship) appears impossible to enforce; whether it would be satisfied would depend on the character of the provider and on whether his or her trustworthiness could be, and was, adequately assessed.

In light of these complications, as well as no doubt others that I have not brought forth, it might reasonably be concluded that gamete donation ought to be legally prohibited on the grounds that it is more likely to fail than to pass moral muster. Yet, because it seems quite unlikely that gamete donation will be legally prohibited; because current practices of gamete donation leave so much to be desired (indeed, they are totally unregulated in most countries and to my mind reprehensible); and, more to the point, because I think that there is in fact a good case for considering gamete donation legitimate *under some circumstances* (roughly outlined above), my own position is that ethical reflection supports the work of legal scholars and legislators seeking to reform, rather than abolish, this practice.[74]

It might be objected that such reforms as I have contemplated would reduce the number of persons willing to provide gametes.[75] To which the reply must be: if the only way to attract providers were to ignore the demands of morality, what could recommend doing so? I agree with Callahan that compassion for persons desiring biologically related children should not overrule *all* other considerations, first and foremost, on the argument that I have developed, procreators' duties of responsibility toward the children whom they have presumed to bring into being.[76]

Another possible though quite different objection to my argument is that it does not demand enough of gamete providers. For gamete donation to be morally legitimate, should not another condition be that (6) the provider agrees to serve as the fallback parent, so to speak, should the intended parent or parents die or prove incompetent? It seems likely that this condition, though well founded in principle, would indeed radically reduce the number of providers, perhaps only to close family members and friends. But, be that as it may, I do not think that this condition is strictly necessary. A solution is to match intended parents with providers only when, first, there is good reason to think that the intended parents are competent (more or less condition 1 above); second, the intended parents are in good health with a reasonable life expectancy (call this condition 1a); and third, the intended parents have family or close friends who commit to forming a relationship with the child and, should the need arise, assuming parental responsibilities and rights toward him or her (call this condition 1b). In this case, it would more than likely be in the child's interest to be raised by the family or friends rather than the provider.[77]

It might also be wondered whether my argument does not have implications for adoption. In particular, should a parent who gives up a child for adoption be understood to retain some measure of inalienable, nontransferrable obligations toward that child? For example, should the parent have to make available all relevant medical information (condition 2); should the parent be available him or herself if the child has a special medical need that the parent is specially placed to help with (condition 3); should the parent be obligated to have his or her identity revealed when the child comes of age (condition 4); and should the parent have to agree to meet with the child at that point and develop an appropriate relationship (condition 5)? In principle, the answer to all these questions is yes, the parent should; but, as Shiffrin has remarked, "it may facilitate adoptions that promote the child's best interests to waive" the obligations of birth parents.[78] Otherwise, unfit parents might be reluctant to relinquish custody. By contrast, should such obligations deter gamete providers, no harm will be done to nonexistent, merely potential children, and the potential of harm to children born of irresponsible providers will have been avoided.

Before turning to surrogacy, a word is appropriate about the responsibilities of clinicians et al., lest they be forgotten. As I have explained, on the causal account, they too incur procreative costs. To the objection that this position is absurd, Dr. Frankenstein serves as a standing rejoinder (see the conclusion of §2). In the normal case, however, there seems little reason to hold that clinicians et al. do wrong in alienating parental obligations, or in other words (less offensive to our linguistic sensibilities) allowing others to pick up the procreative costs. So long as the clinicians et al. have good reason to believe that the intended parent or parents will fulfill their obligations, and the clinicians et al. do their work competently (for example: screening providers for disease and exercising care in fertilizing an egg in vitro and transferring a zygote), then helping others realize the great good of having a child appears as ample justification for stepping aside, rather than potentially interfering with the development of intimate parent-child bonds, which require a significant measure of privacy.[79] In other words, so long as a child is entrusted to good parents, and was not somehow harmed by clinicians' recklessness, proportionate reason warrants clearing clinicians et. al of any further duties. Gamete providers, by contrast, have more to answer for. Unlike clinicians and technicians, gamete providers make, in a sense, a "gift of self" toward the child-to-be in providing semen or eggs.[80] To put the same point in different terms, they not only *effect* the child, but *affect* him or her genetically.

The debate over surrogacy, more precisely commercial surrogacy, is complicated by the further question, which I have not addressed though I have adverted to it here and there, of whether "women's labor" is rightly treated as a commodity. (The question is put forcefully by Elizabeth Anderson, to whom I have referred several times.) If we put this question aside—though we must return to it—the case for the legitimacy of surrogacy, *under some circumstances*, appears as strong as the case for gamete donation, under the same circumstances, the necessary changes having been made. (Substitute the word 'surrogate' for 'gamete provider' in my list of five conditions.) An interesting question here, however, is whether a gestational surrogate ought to be held to the fourth and fifth conditions: namely, to have her identity revealed when the child comes of age, should the child not know it already, and to meet with the child at that point, should he or she seek to meet, and to develop with him or her an appropriate relationship, again should the child so wish. Given the importance, however it is to be qualified, of genetics in our constitution and identity, we can understand why a child in search of self-definition might want to meet with his or her genetic parents. But would a child have similarly pressing reasons to want to meet with his or her gestational surrogate? Wittgenstein's remark that what is distinctive to a philosophical problem is that *we do not know our way about* with it seems appropriate here, despite the quite different context.[81] When it is a question of how a child will feel toward and think about his or her gestational surrogate, we do not know our way about—and so it seems better to err on the side of asking for more from surrogates rather than less.

Should my five conditions be satisfied, it appears possible for at least noncommercial surrogacy to pass moral muster, though human nature is surely known well enough to anticipate that such arrangements—say a sister or a cousin agrees to bear a child for a couple—might prove deeply fraught. In other words, it is not a foregone conclusion that noncommercial surrogacy arrangements will in all cases satisfy the criteria of proportionate reason, perhaps in particular the third criterion, paraphrasing somewhat, that (c) the manner of pursuing the good of family not ultimately undermine this good (should, for example, the child's birth lead to the fraying of relationships, or significant confusion and conflict for the child as he or she ages).

Put significant sums of money into the mix—in other words, return the focus to *commercial* surrogacy—and we need to think again about whether surrogacy satisfies the criteria of proportionate reason. As the New Jersey Supreme Court stated in the Baby M case, with tens of thousands of dollars at stake (most of that money going to surrogate brokers), commercial surrogacy arrangements court the risk that the profit motive will predominate, permeate, and ultimately govern the transaction,[82] to the detriment of both the surrogate and the child. The danger to the child here is that the intended parent or parents may prove wealthy but unfit.[83] This danger can be addressed by regulation mandating, as one legal scholar has proposed, "some form of pre-birth judicial review to insure that a child born to a surrogate is given to the custody of persons who meet minimum standards of fitness for parenthood."[84] The potential harm to the surrogate, which is not as apparent, appears less amenable to a regulatory solution—unless this solution were to ban commercial surrogacy contracts altogether and to subject brokers who arrange such contracts to criminal penalties. Presently, both in the United States and globally, laws concerning commercial surrogacy vary significantly.[85]

Here, in brief, is Anderson's case against treating women's labor as a commodity, which is to say a good that is properly subject to the norms of the market, which she emphatically states women's labor "*is not.*"[86] The key point is that "[p]regnancy is not simply a biological process but also a social practice"—the norms of which aim to foster deep bonds of affection between the pregnant woman and developing child.[87] (For simplicity's sake, just think how strangers may congratulate a pregnant woman and ask when she is due.) The problem is not that the practice of surrogacy threatens "to remake pregnancy into a form of drudgery" and thereby to wreak systemic consequences on the bond between mothers and children, though sometimes Anderson does appear to gravitate toward this sort of claim.[88] Instead, more precisely, the problem is that, "*unless* we were to remake pregnancy into a form of drudgery" (emphasis added), we can expect that at least some women who are engaged as surrogates will develop what Anderson terms "the precious emotional ties which the mother may rightly and properly establish with her 'product,' the child."[89] From the point of view of the market, however, "the woman's transformation of moral and emotional perspective . . . looks like a capricious and selfish exercise of will."[90] In other words, it appears wrong that the surrogate has developed such emotional ties: she has not done "right and proper" in becoming attached to the child; she ought to have repressed, as illegitimate because against the terms of the surrogacy contract, whatever feelings of love she came to have. For her love was sold before it ever came to pass. But, to reiterate, "*unless* we were to remake pregnancy into a form of drudgery"—unless the social practices surrounding pregnancy were to be transformed so that they did *not* encourage moral and emotional transformation on the part of pregnant women during what is, physiologically and psychologically, a period of upheaval[91]—surrogacy contracts practically invite abuse of surrogates. Lest a surrogate become deeply attached to the child, her thoughts and feelings must be vigilantly policed and, if necessary, disciplined and even manipulated; whatever love she comes to feel, if it shows signs of intensity, must be denigrated and denied legitimacy; and finally she herself must be treated as a commodity, a good properly subject to market norms, rather than a person whose emotional relations with others warrant consideration and whose autonomy demands protection.[92]

Imagine for a moment that you are a surrogate broker. Anderson's case against your business is simple. Your financial interest in making sure that the surrogate surrenders the baby (otherwise you make no money) makes it likely that, in cases where the surrogate begins to bond with the baby and shows signs of not wanting to part with him or her, you will (1) not honor her autonomy, but manipulate her to do what you want, namely, surrender the baby; (2) fail to show sensitive regard for her emotions, but try to make her feel bad about even thinking of emotionally devastating the contracting parents; and (3) treat her as a mere means to your end of making money.

To be clear, the argument here is not that, as the Baby M judgment declared, the surrogate mother "never makes a totally voluntary, informed decision, for quite clearly any decision prior to the baby's birth is, in the most important sense, uninformed, and any decision after that, compelled by a pre-existing contractual commitment, the threat of a lawsuit, and the inducement of a [significant] payment, is less than totally voluntary."[93] As Lori Andrews has remarked in opposition to such a claim, given surrogacy contracts' myriad riders and the volumes of publicity after the Baby M case, it is reasonable to hold that the decision of any surrogate should now be informed. What's more (to speak for a moment like a legal brief), (1) the legal doctrine of informed consent does not, in any event, presuppose "that one must have the experience first before one can make an informed judgment about whether to agree to the experience"; (2) the argument that a woman's hormonal changes during pregnancy make it impossible for her to predict in advance the consequences of her relinquishment "is a dangerous one for feminists to make"; and finally (3) the record of women who have been surrogates does not support the claim that surrogacy invariably involves economic exploitation (though of course it might, as critics have worried about the "outsourcing" of surrogacy to countries such as India).[94]

I think that Andrews is right on each of these points; none, however, counters Anderson's claim that treating women's labor as a commodity practically invites the mistreatment of surrogates. To be sure, any given arrangement might go fine: the surrogate might suffer neither trauma nor abuse. But the point is that surrogacy contracts create the conditions for abuse, whether it comes to pass or not. It might be proposed that a solution to this danger is simply to make surrogacy contracts legally unenforceable, or to reform the contracts, along the lines of adoption, "to respect a change of mind of a biological parent within some specified time period."[95] Anderson's counters to these proposals seem to me right: first, "there is no feasible way to prevent brokers from bullying and exploiting mothers in a regime that holds such contracts legal but unenforceable";[96] second, "granting the surrogate mother the option to reserve her parental rights after birth . . . would pressure the [contracting] agency to demean the mother's self-regard more than ever."[97] The upshot is that the practice of commercial surrogacy appears not to satisfy the criteria of proportionate reason, in particular the first and second criteria (negatively stated) that (a) a lesser value is not preferred to a greater one and that (b) evil is not unnecessarily caused. Yes, having a child is a great good, but it is not so great that existent persons (namely, women engaged as surrogates) may be subject to abuse so that a not-yet-existent person might be brought into being. Further, there are other ways of having a child, among which adoption, that appear less apt to cause evil than commercial surrogacy is. In brief then, though commercial surrogates may be able to keep faith with the children to be born, a legal system that professes to do right by persons cannot, in good faith, countenance commercial surrogacy.

A final objection to Anderson's argument deserves to be addressed. It might well be asked whether there are not other lines of work in which people have to police their thoughts and feelings: for example, soldiers in battle, judges in courts, doctors conducting intimate examinations on patients, etc. Vigilant policing of thoughts and feelings is entirely appropriate in these cases—but defenders of commercial surrogacy might say exactly the same of the surrogate. After all, she signed up for the job. Where lies the difference between the surrogate and, say, the soldier who enlisted for financial reasons and then, in battle, must police his thoughts and feelings? I think that the answer must be that it is part of the practice—constitutive of the role—of being a soldier, judge, or doctor to police one's thoughts and feelings in particular ways. It might be claimed that doing so is likewise part of the practice—constitutive of the role—of being a surrogate; but the surrogate, as a pregnant woman, also has a part, so to speak, in broader and deeper social practices that we have good reason to value and that run precisely counter to and work against what is demanded of her as a surrogate. And I take this point to be the heart of Anderson's objection to commercial surrogacy.

There ends my engagement with the practices of gamete donation and surrogacy and my defense of the causal account against the charge that it is useless in the assignment of parental responsibility when new reproductive technologies are employed. A more general objection, however, ought to be anticipated; it can also, I think, be quickly dispatched, though I do not deny its pertinence. The objection is that we typically would not contemplate interferences with procreative liberty in cases of what might be called traditional procreation—that is, when reproductive technologies are not employed. What warrants, then, such interferences when reproductive technologies are employed?

What is lacking about this objection is that it does not identify the reason why we typically would not contemplate interference in the normal case. I propose that the reason is this: if the state had the power to prevent reproduction by ordinary means, there is little power that the state would not have. Giving the state such power would mean the end of any public-private distinction. The state's power would encompass our bodies and extend over the most intimate domains of our formerly "private" lives. Whatever else is objectionable about such a proposal—Hugh LaFollette's notorious paper "Licensing Parents" is required reading in this regard[98]—it likely would prove disastrous in all but the most ideal of states.[99] By contrast, as Rebecca Dresser has noted, "[b]y enlisting outsiders to assist them in having children, people constructing surrogacy agreements [or turning to gamete donation] remove reproduction from the private realm" of sexual activity.[100] Accordingly, regulation of such reproductive arrangements need not involve any objectionable invasions of personal liberties. Instead, regulations may be constructed with an eye toward protecting the vulnerable.

In the next chapter, I turn to the ethics of prenatal genetic enhancement, where again there is reason to be concerned about protecting the vulnerable.

5 Good Enough Parenting?
The Child's Right to an Open Future
and the Ethics of Prenatal Genetic
Enhancement

The majority opinion in the U.S. Supreme Court case of *Wisconsin v. Yoder* (406 U.S. 205 [1972]) provoked philosophical commentary that is remarkable for its passion and conviction. There are, occasionally, even hints of outrage, which the subject of other people's children will for some reason elicit. As is well known, the Court found that Old Order Amish parents who had declined, in violation of Wisconsin law, to send their children to school beyond the eighth grade were exempted from compliance under the Free Exercise Clause of the First Amendment. In response, Kenneth Henley wrote:

> It might be claimed that some traditional ways of life—for instance, that of the Amish—could not survive the requirement that older children be allowed to go to school with children from the larger community and to learn about science and technology. *If* this claim is true, then such traditional ways of life have no right to survive, for their survival is at the expense of the liberty of the children who are born into them.[1]

Joel Feinberg was little less strident in a paper that has become a classic in the children's rights literature, "The Child's Right to an Open Future." According to him, "From the philosophical standpoint," in "the technologically complex modern world," an "educable youth whose parents legally withdraw him from school has suffered an invasion of his rights in trust" whether he is fourteen (the age of the children in *Yoder*) or sixteen (the age to which Wisconsin's law required school attendance).[2]

This chapter is concerned, as its subtitle indicates, with the ethics of prenatal genetic enhancement. I approach this question here, however, not directly but by examining first the arguments made by Henley and Feinberg, among others, that children's "anticipatory autonomy rights"—rights to choose freely among various ways of life, in particular with respect to vocation and religion—must be preserved throughout childhood. It is no part of my purpose to dispute that there are rightly limits to parental power. I take it for granted that, since children are persons, albeit immature, of course there should be limits; and of course, by way of example, the Roman magistrates and people were wrong to stand idly by as Cassius threw his son, the demagogic Spurius Cassius, to his death—a favorite example of Sir Robert Filmer's showing, to his mind, the rightful power of a father over his children,[3] but perhaps instead why we should be grateful that the Roman republic and then empire gave way.[4] My dispute is with the way that the so-called "liberal argument" (Amy Gutmann's term) goes about setting these limits to parental power: namely, in John Rawls's language, by making the concept of the right prior to that of the good.[5]

This sort of argument has become dominant in bioethics. In discussions of the genetic enhancement of children, the demand that the child's right to an open future be preserved functions not only to restrict what parents may rightly do, but to legitimate parental action so long as this demand is satisfied. In brief, I argue in the following that focusing in this way on the child's right to an open future truncates the thinking that we need to do about the brave new world that biotechnology may be calling into being.[6] Proponents of the child's right to an open future would no doubt acknowledge that the so-called good enough parent does more than respect his or her child's anticipatory autonomy rights; but it is too little considered in the literature—though the question has by no means been simply overlooked—whether changes in the ways of becoming a parent could put the normative unconditionality of the parent-child relationship at risk. My concern in the following, simply put, is that attention to rights not blind us to implications for goods.

I now go on at some length to consider the grounds and limits of parental power with respect to the *education* of children. I ask the reader to remember, however, that my interest in this inquiry is to gain insight into what a parent owes his or her children. What I seek to establish, to be clear, is that preserving a child's right to an open future is not "good enough" to legitimate the genetic enhancement of children. My main claim is that, in the so-called liberal argument I go on to criticize, concern for the child's *future* autonomy figures too largely. Whether the Amish, by contrast, get autonomy right is a further question that I do not pretend to answer, though I am sympathetic to critics who suggest we should say no. If the Amish have a failing in this regard, however, it looks to be a failing to respect the child's *present* autonomy—a point to which I return.

§1. THE "LIBERAL ARGUMENT"

The problem of children's rights in liberal constitutional democracies is nicely summed up in the famous first sentence of the opening chapter of Rousseau's *Social Contract*: "Man is born free, and everywhere he is in chains."[7] This claim would have given the seventeenth-century monarchist

Robert Filmer fits: it is the first principle of his political thought, against which Locke developed his own, that no person is born free, but from the beginning into subjection to his or her father. (We have Hobbes to thank, of all people, for making the case for the mother.[8]) And Filmer has a point: children may be "born to" freedom and equality, as Locke countered,[9] but it is nevertheless true they need to be swaddled when they are born, and that they are then subject to parental rule for years to come. So, if we look around, we see children everywhere in chains: fastened into strollers and car seats; caged in cribs and play pens; taken and in some instances dragged to church, synagogue, or mosque; enrolled in school; and, in the fighting words of one critic of religious education, even indoctrinated into parents' "value systems."[10]

It is a good question what justifies parental authority. It is also an old question, reaching back to arguments over the binding power of the Sinai covenant on the children and children's children of the Israelites who stood at the foot of the mountain.[11] For Filmer, the answer was "generation"; but, as Locke scathingly observed, "He that should demand of him [namely, Filmer], How, or for what Reason it is, that begetting a Child gives the Father such an Absolute Power over him, will find him answer nothing."[12] Hobbes, remarkably, claimed that parental right of dominion was derived not from generation, "but from the child's consent, either express or by sufficient other arguments declared," among which he apparently counted breastfeeding.[13] Yet it is doubtful, to say the least, that children, and especially infants, can give consent to parental dominion in any meaningful sense.[14] What's more, as Gutmann observes, "many things [parents] do to [children] are perfectly acceptable even when they explicitly refuse consent":[15] take, for example, brushing their teeth, coercing them into eating their vegetables, or giving them "time out," if not sending them to their rooms or some other means of punishment, when all else fails. So it appears that grounding parental authority in children's consent will not do. Locke realized as much and made a critical move: he derived parents' rights from the parents' duty "to take care of their Off-spring, during the imperfect state of Childhood."[16] In his hands, what he called parental "right of *Tuition*" becomes "rather the Priviledge [*sic*] of Children, and Duty of Parents, than any Prerogative of Paternal Power."[17] In other words, parental authority both arises from and is circumscribed by children's interests, which it is premised children cannot be entrusted either to understand or to pursue until they reach the age of reason or, in contemporary philosophical language, until they develop "the full-fledged moral agency required for full citizenship in the moral community."[18]

Locke's account has more or less carried the day,[19] and I follow him in thinking that parental rights are grounded in and derived from parental responsibilities (though it is certainly intelligible that one might have some measure of responsibilities, yet only limited rights or no rights at all).[20] It is now commonly assumed in the philosophical literature and in the public practice of liberal constitutional democracies that "parental rights are nothing like property rights," and that they "derive [instead] from the fact that children are often incapable of effectively exercising their rights and making rational [that is, well-informed] decisions about their interests."[21] The parent-child relationship is cast as a "stewardship" relationship—not quite a fiduciary or trustee relationship, from which there are subtle differences[22]—with the parent empowered to exercise discretion and authority in defense and pursuit of the child's interests. The obvious question is how to specify these interests. Here begins my argument with the literature.

There appear to be two problems in trying to specify these interests: first, children cannot be taken as authorities on this matter (again, it is premised that they are "often incapable of . . . making rational decisions about their interests"); second, parents have only limited information about the future self of the child whose interests they are charged to protect and promote. For who knows what projects, values, and commitments he or she will come to have (or even, nowadays, whether he will choose to become she or she he)? Robert Noggle accordingly observes that "[t]he situation parents face is structurally similar to that of the contractor in Rawls's Original Position: both must protect and promote the interests of someone whose particular goals, concerns, attachments, and values they do not know." What is needed, Noggle goes on to propose, is a "'parental veil of ignorance' that hides the particulars of the future adult self whose interests the parent is to protect and promote."[23] Gutmann agrees, and recommends "Rawls's primary good standard" as the proper guide for parents' decisions.[24] To quote from *A Theory of Justice*:

> Paternalistic decisions are to be guided by the individual's own settled preferences and interests insofar as these are rational, or failing a knowledge of these, by the theory of primary goods. As we know less and less about a person, we [should] act for him as we would act for ourselves from the standpoint of the original position. We [should] try to get for him the things he presumably wants whatever else he wants

—which is just what primary goods are on Rawls's account: goods that "normally have a use whatever a person's rational plan of life."[25] In brief, then, according to Gutmann, parents should seek to ensure their children "the greatest range of reasonable choice . . . as adults."[26] Providing children primary goods is the means to this end.

We might well question, however, the claim that parents have only limited information about the future self of the child. There is a sense in which this claim is obviously true, but the claim can also be taken too far, such that it becomes tendentious if not nonsensical. Yes, it is true that parents cannot predict the future, and parents' power to determine outcomes should not be exaggerated; but it is also true that "[w]hether a certain sort of life would please a child often depends upon *how* he has been socialized,"[27] and parents' power to determine outcomes should not be underestimated, either. The so-called liberal argument as I have presented it to this point fails to make clear why parents must step behind the veil of ignorance. After all, who is better placed to identify, and then to encourage or amend, a child's emerging interests and traits! To repeat: yes, parents cannot know for sure just how their child will turn out, but as a matter of fact they can do much to shape him or her, which is just what motivates the criticism of *Yoder* and the call to preserve the child's right to an open future to begin with. Feinberg claims that children's future liberties of choice as adults "must be protected now (in advance)," which according to him requires that parents' claims to raise their children as they will (in *Yoder*, to become members of a separatist religious community) "must retreat before the claims of children that they be permitted to reach maturity with as many open options, opportunities, and advantages as possible."[28]

Gutmann has developed the "liberal argument" thoroughly. Recall her claim that parents should seek to ensure their children "the greatest range of reasonable choice . . . as adults." Why? The answer that parents have only limited information about the future self of the child distracts from what is really at issue. What we need to know is why parents would do wrong to seek to shape their children so that, for example, they would have "no realistic prospect of pursuing a lifestyle radically opposed to Amish values."[29] Put positively, we need to know why parents have an obligation to raise their children to be autonomous: as this term is glossed in the literature, to be capable of critically assessing and revising their own conception of the good, and then of effectively choosing among a range of feasible and valuable options.[30]

Here is how Gutmann answers. For her, what is really at stake is justice to children; her basic theory of justice is Rawls's. First, she relativizes the concept of a primary good. They are not, for her, "timeless or universal," but "reflect a common understanding within a society of what goods rational individuals, ignorant of their particular interests, would want provided for them within that society."[31] It follows that the goods that parents are obligated to provide children will vary with and be "dependent upon the nature of the society within which children are to be raised."[32] What is critical in this regard is the given society's "common understanding" of the goods that all rational individuals presumably want whatever else they want. Now, as what Gutmann calls "our society" offers and values "a broad range of choices to its adult members" among conceptions of the good life, the upshot for her is that "parents have an obligation to allow their children to be exposed to the choices available in their extrafamilial society."[33] More strongly, the upshot is that children must be educated so that they will be capable of "choosing competently among a broad range of conceptions of the good life," as this competence is, according to Gutmann, commonly understood as a "fundamental good" in liberal societies like ours (though whether *more* choice really is always good is open to doubt).[34] In sum, "The content of children's right to education will depend upon what is adequate for living a full life within their society."[35] Stipulate that it is the common understanding in our society that a full life requires freedom of choice among multiple conceptions of the good life, and the case is closed. But I hope it is clear that the fix was in from the start, and that all too much rides on stipulation of what "our society" (whatever that is) holds dear.[36] Gutmann simply deprives the Amish of a voice. In her hands, Amish society is swallowed up by greater American society.[37] Otherwise her procedure would not yield the decision that she wants. (By the way, social scientists who have studied the Amish doubt that most Amish children enjoy such "entirely free choice, because Amish socialization funnels youth toward church membership" by thorough immersion "in a total ethnic world with its own language, symbols, and world view."[38])

At the bottom of the so-called liberal argument, once we put aside all the talk of our society's putatively common understanding, what we find is the passionate conviction that the absolute freedom that children are born with—recall Rousseau—must be essentially preserved throughout childhood. What chains are necessary to bring children from the state of nature to civil society must break of themselves, without trauma, once children come of age.[39] It might sound ideal; but I think it is worth wondering here, with Michael Sandel, whether a person who is so unencumbered is not "an ideally free and rational agent, but [instead] a person wholly without character, without moral depth," all too free from the claims of conscience.[40]

§2. THE GOOD AND THE RIGHT

At this point, and after these fighting words of my own, proponents of the so-called liberal argument might be moved to retort, well, what then is your solution? For surely you don't believe that anything goes; more concretely, surely you don't believe that children may rightly be deprived of education altogether, say as Huck Finn's Pap sought to deprive Huck lest he prove better than his family.[41] To ratchet up the stakes and make her case more compelling, Gutmann remarks that

> [p]erhaps the stakes in the Yoder case were too small to impress the dilemma it posed upon us; only one or two years of compulsory schooling were in dispute. But imagine if another well-established religious group otherwise identical to the Amish were to forbid *all*

formal education for their children for the same reasons that the Amish prohibit schooling beyond the eighth grade.[42]

She also notes that Justice Byron White wrote in his concurring opinion in *Yoder* that "[t]his would be a very different case for me if respondent's claim were that their religion forbade their children from attending any school at any time and from complying in any way with the educational standards set by the State."[43] Gutmann comments: "The Court's decision might have differed, but the rights at issue remain the same"[44]—implying, if I understand correctly, that logically the *Yoder* case ought to have been decided the same as the hypothetical case in question. In other words, Gutmann appears to hold that, while depriving a child of education altogether is surely worse than depriving a child of an education that seeks to prepare him or her for "living a full life within [our] society," both courses of action ought to be criticized for the same basic reason: the child is deprived of his or her due as a person; justice is not served.

In keeping with this view, proponents of the so-called liberal argument object to Chief Justice Warren Burger's statement in his majority opinion in *Yoder* that

> [i]t is one thing to say that compulsory education for a year or two beyond the eighth grade may be necessary when its goal is the preparation of the child for life in modern society as the majority live, but it is quite another if the goal of education be viewed as the preparation of the child for life in the separated agrarian community that is the keystone of the Amish faith.[45]

Feinberg asks in opposition, "But how is the 'goal of education' to be viewed?" and answers, as we have seen already, that education should "send [the child] out into the adult world with as many open opportunities as possible."[46] This is, however, precisely to say that education should prepare the child "for life in modern society," since the opportunities that Feinberg has in mind—engineer, research scientist, lawyer, business executive—are all opportunities within modern society.[47] From this perspective, to deprive a child of an education adequate for "living a full life within [our] society" is little better than depriving a child of an education altogether. In both cases, many options will be irrevocably foreclosed, and so, to quote Feinberg again, "critical life decisions will have been made irreversibly for a person well before he reaches the age of full discretion when he should be expected, in a free society, to make them himself."[48]

The way to respond to this challenge is to articulate a different conception of the goal of education and of a child's interest in becoming educated. To answer fully would be, to say the least, a rather big undertaking,[49] so I limit myself here to articulating only a piece of the answer.

It makes sense that education should serve socialization (though not only socialization): surely a child has an interest in becoming a well-functioning adult. To this end, she needs to acquire fundamental skills, such as basic literacy. Children have not only cognitive needs, however, but profound physical and emotional needs. These can be fulfilled, as Shelley Burtt has observed, along *many* pathways,[50] though it hardly needs reminding that much can also go wrong, and even terribly wrong. In any event, it makes sense to hold, as Burtt puts it, that "the state can and ought to demand of parents that they fulfill in some reasonable way children's developmental needs."[51] To deprive a child of all formal education would be to do her a wrong inasmuch as her interest in becoming a well-functioning adult would be disregarded. But does a child have an interest, as the so-called liberal argument would have it, in entering "the adult world with as many open opportunities as possible," or in any event (and more intelligibly) with "at least a reasonable range of the skills and capacities necessary to provide [her] the choice of a reasonable array of different life plans available to members of [her] society"?[52]

I propose that the answer is a qualified *yes*: yes, the child does have an interest in having a reasonable range of skills and capacities in order to choose from a reasonable array of different life plans—but the critical question is *what society* she is to be educated to live within and whether education for life within this society may be expected to fulfill in some reasonable way the child's primary developmental needs (physical, emotional, cognitive).[53] What counts as a reasonable range of skills and capacities and a reasonable array of different life plans will vary from society to society according to each society's form of life, so asking whether this or that range or array is "reasonable" makes no sense in the abstract. What we need to focus on first and foremost, then, is more basic: again, whether the way that a child will be raised may be expected to fulfill his or her primary needs. For the child's fundamental interest is to be educated in such a way that she can have a good human life, not just or principally "open," and it is not the case that having "as many open opportunities as possible" is necessary to a good life, however much such openness might be valued in our times.[54] Admittedly, a child born into a relatively self-sufficient society that is itself within a greater society, like a state, would need to be assured a realistic right of exit into this greater society in which she is a citizen. And, in a liberal constitutional democracy, she would also need to be educated to be capable of adequately fulfilling her duties as a citizen.[55] Yet, provided that the child is educated in such a way that she develops her basic capacities, the demand that she have a right to exit is surely satisfied: should she leave, she would be able to lead a decent life—and she could always go for her general equivalency degree. So too is the demand that she be capable of responsible citizenship, even if she will not please so-called strong participatory democrats in the tradition of Rousseau's republicanism.[56] The majority opinion in *Yoder* may be read as finding that Amish education serves the normal development of basic human capacities,[57] and that worries about the right of exit and civic responsibility are then misplaced.[58]

Proponents of the so-called liberal argument, and critics of the Court's decision, nonetheless see educating a child for life in Amish society as unduly restrictive. For these critics, such an education does not serve justice. Perhaps they would concede that such a life could be a good human life, but this question never arises in the literature that I have discussed, which totally ignores social scientific studies of the Amish. The priority of the right to the good renders irrelevant the question of whether the Amish life could reasonably be understood as a good life.

The so-called liberal argument may also be criticized for distorting the liberal tradition (hence my use of the qualification "so-called" throughout this chapter). As William Galston has observed in an oft-cited paper, when "we inspect the liberal philosophical tradition, there emerge two quite different strands of liberal thought based on two distinct principles," namely, autonomy or self-direction, on the one hand; and diversity or toleration of differences among individuals and groups, on the other.[59] Looking to history and in particular back to the Reformation, Galston claims that "properly understood, liberalism is about the protection of diversity, not the valorization of choice," and notes that "[t]o place an ideal of autonomous choice . . . at the core of liberalism is in fact to narrow the range of possibilities available within liberal societies."[60] As we have seen, proponents of the so-called liberal argument say to this last charge, So much the worse for traditional ways of life; but this answer would have been astonishing to the Anabaptists, among others, who came to the New World seeking religious freedom for themselves, their children, and their children's children. And so it makes sense to wonder who has the liberal tradition right.

Before moving on to the ethics of prenatal genetic enhancement, consider this brief dialogue, for which I draw principally from the sociologist Donald Kraybill's *The Riddle of Amish Culture*:

ENGLISH (which is what the Amish typically call non-Amish people): "By what right do [you] Amish parents limit the education of [your] children, restrict occupational choice, cap opportunities for personal achievement, stifle artistic expression, and prescribe rigid sex roles? . . . Denying [your] youth education makes a mockery of modern justice. Would it not only be fair . . . if [your] children were required to attend at least several years of public high school to taste the fruits of progress? Then they would be free to pursue professional careers or return to Amish life."

AMISH: "By what right . . . do [you English] parents push [your] children through the turnstiles of modernity, to face incessant choices that carry heavy emotional loads? By what right do [you] deprive [your] youth of the psychological security and personal identity that come from membership in a lasting and durable group? In fact . . ., should not [your] youth be required to live several years in a traditional community to experience communal life firsthand?"[61] And it's also worth asking (to make the Amish speak now in the voice of a contemporary philosopher) "to *what* does the mind open when all goes as [you English hold that] it should. A commonly assumed answer among [you] seems to be that we need not bother much with the question. Once we liberate our children . . . by exposing them to the diversity around them and encouraging them to think for themselves, then all will be well. That would make sense [though] only if the diversity that abounded around them really were an edifying ethical pluralism." But "[w]hat exposure to diversity really amounts to is very often something" quite different, namely, induction into a consumer culture that is destructive of all higher purposes.[62] So please: no more talk of your justice. And God save us from your high schools.

§3. GOOD ENOUGH?

As I remarked in this chapter's introduction, in discussions of the ethics of prenatal genetic enhancement, the demand that the child's right to an open future be preserved functions not only to restrict what parents may rightly do, but to legitimate parental action so long as this demand is satisfied. This is the argument made by advocates of so-called liberal eugenics.[63] As one oft-cited text puts it:

> Recognizing the right to an open future is compatible with according substantial discretion to parents to use genetic interventions, just as they would other environmental interventions, to attempt to give their children what they might consider to be the best life possible. What is required is that those interventions do not so narrow children's range of opportunities as to violate their right to an open future.[64]

Or as another author puts it, "capacity-enhancement" must be "neutral between a wide range of life plans and suboptimal with respect to any particular one."[65] This author goes on to propose a Rawls-inspired "maximin constraint on capacity enhancement," namely, "Goods of genetic engineering must be allocated to an individual in a way that improves prospects associated with all possible life plans—most especially the worst off life plan," which is to say the life plan a child's *parents* might consider least desirable for her.[66] For "[t]he aim is to equip the person-to-be no matter what life plan she opts for."[67] Permissible genetic interventions will then be those that improve "prospects associated with all life plans"; impermissible genetic interventions will be those that unduly restrict a person's choice of life plan. What is critical is that a child's parents keep his or her future "open."[68]

Now, I agree that an important distinction has to be drawn between enhancements that "support a rather wide range of plans" and those that will be "plan specific."[69] Moreover, I share the objection to plan-specific capacities that they potentially limit "the liberty of the prospective offspring."[70] The danger is that there might prove to be "a mismatch between capacities and life plans," a possibility that can never be ruled out given the "asymmetry in the way a person's goals on the one hand, and that same person's capacities on the other, can be influenced by genetic engineering." (It is assumed that goals generally cannot be engineered—"[n]o amount of information is likely to enable us to pair genotypes with life plans"[71]—whereas the capacities, per hypothesis, can.) If there were such a mismatch between capacities and life plan, the child might grow to feel locked into a life for which she has no passion, or fated to a life plan chosen by somebody else.[72] This sort of worry is what leads proponents of liberal eugenics to appeal to the child's right to an open future.

But consider this simple example: a child who has been genetically enhanced to have extraordinary musical talents. Admittedly, her genetic makeup does not determine that she *must* live her life in one preset way, or that she cannot flourish in different, unforeseen ways. Given the importance of environmental factors in a person's development, she might not even have any outstanding capacity for music.[73] So not only have her interests not been harmed by her having been brought into being as she is (for the sake of the argument, the only way that she could have been), but her right to an open future does not appear to have been violated. What needs to be considered, however, is that her parents obviously had high expectations for her. Even John Robertson, a great proponent of reproductive liberty, allows that "parents might have unrealistic expectations of children who have been subject to efforts to make them superior." Yet he puts hope, rather incredibly, in "expert counseling and preparation to minimize" any dangers.[74] With this help, parents who turned to genetic manipulation "out of love and concern for the child's welfare" could learn to allow the adolescent in question to discover and develop her personality with the same freedom as any other young person. But it is an awfully pretty story, and certainly not to be expected in all cases, which may be to say only the least.[75] Conflict, or at least disappointment, seems more likely.

New reproductive technologies on the horizon promise (realistically or not) parental choice of children's genetic characteristics. Consider the titles of two of the more influential texts in Anglo-American bioethics defending the use of new reproductive technologies: Robertson's *Children of Choice: Freedom and the New Reproductive Technologies*; and Allen Buchanan, Dan Brock, Norman Daniels, and Daniel Wikler's *From Chance to Choice: Genetics and Justice*. As I noted in this chapter's introduction, what authors who defend these technologies often leave unexamined is whether parents' choosing the sort of child they want risks compromising the normative unconditionality of the parent-child relationship by rendering the parents' love for the child all too conditional: namely, on the child's satisfying parental expectations. In other words, authors who defend these technologies often fail to examine whether the use of these technologies might conflict with, and even work against, a basic, if "imperfect" parental obligation to meet a child's primary emotional needs though developing an affective relationship with him or her—in the language of chapter 2, a deep parent-child bond that has the power to help reconcile a child to the fact and conditions of his or her existence, and make the child's life one that he or she has reason to affirm.[76]

We need to consider if the concern in question is well founded. In other words, is it supported by any evidence or data? Three sorts of objections can be anticipated. One is that it is difficult to see reason to worry about at least some, if not all, of the enhancements that proponents of liberal eugenics have in view. For example, what risk would be run by enhancements of the human immune system; increases in attention, alertness, and the speed with which information is processed by the brain; and improvements in memory?[77] Or, for that matter, what risk would be run by giving a child perfect pitch, if this capacity could ever be programmed genetically? Would such enhancements really run the risk of compromising the normative unconditionality of the parent-child relationship? It is difficult to see how.

A second objection is that it is in fact part of the role of parent to seek to "enhance" one's children, and parents have been doing it for millennia in all kinds of innovative ways. Moreover, as Dan Brock has observed, the attempt to shape children's development not only is "not incompatible with parents' unconditional love and acceptance of their children," but more often is an expression of this love.[78] Accordingly, we typically do not criticize but praise the parent who provides his or her child a fine education, tutors, lessons, special camps, and so forth.[79] These are, admittedly, so-called environmental rather than genetic "interventions," but they can be similarly effective to the genetic interventions in question, and can have similarly irrevocable effects on the child. In this regard, what is the difference, morally speaking, between giving a child a vaccination after birth and genetically enhancing his or her immune system before birth? These considerations lend credence to the claim that there is a strong argument from precedent for judging permissible at least some kinds of genetic enhancements.

Third and last, the concern that I have raised might be dismissed as baseless. Brock has speculated that, since "unconditional love and acceptance of children by their parents is common across a wide range of social conditions and historical periods," it may be genetically programmed, and so can be expected to survive despite new ways of becoming a parent.[80] He has also noted that, if and when genetic enhancement becomes practicable, "[a]ll the experiences of pregnancy, infancy, and early childhood that now develop strong unconditional bonds of love and attachment of parents to their children would [presumably] still take place," and so we could expect parents to go on loving their children unconditionally whether a proclivity to do so is genetically programmed or not.[81] Brock has been joined in this defense by Frances Kamm. In response to Michael Sandel, who has raised concerns like mine,[82] Kamm has asked why, before a child's birth, *caring to have* a child with specific traits or capacities (or, for that matter, without specific disabilities) necessarily implies that one would not *care about* the child, after birth, should he or she turn out not to have the traits or capacities that one sought (or, again for that matter, should he or she turn out to have the disabilities that one wished to avoid).[83] Kamm acknowledges the possibility, even likelihood of disappointment with such an outcome, but claims that the "source" of the disappointment will or at least could be the "lost resources" that one expended to the end of enhancing one's child, not the child him or herself. In Kamm's words, "There may be disappointment for the child when enhancements fail—that one could not bring about something good for it. But that is different from disappointment in the child."[84]

The appropriate reply to all these objections, I think, is of the form "yes, but." Yes, it is difficult to see how enhancements to the human immune system could put at risk the normative unconditionality of the parent-child relationship, as it is likewise difficult to see, at least in the abstract, how increases in attention, alertness, and memory could so the same. Yes, part of the "job" of parenting is to seek to cultivate and to improve one's children so that they might live richer lives, and genetic interventions to this end do not appear radically different in kind from more familiar environmental interventions like tutors and camps.[85] And yes, *caring to have* a child with these or those traits or capacities does not rule out *caring about* the child should he or she turn out differently. After all, the child, at birth, will not be eight-feet tall with the canker of death in its flesh—the child will be no Frankenstein's creature, but a baby much like any other—and so it seems reasonable to think that the parents could well become attached to the child for him or herself, regardless of whether the child exhibits or comes to exhibit the properties that the parents sought to have.

But context matters, and each of these objections, even the third, is remarkably abstract, unruffled by what we can expect and perhaps have to fear from human, all-too-human parents and children in modern consumer cultures characterized, in the social psychologist Barry Schwartz's terms, by "an unequal distribution of scarce and highly desirable commodities."[86]

Yes, caring to have a child who is, say, a boy, or who will be athletic, or who will be mathematically or musically inclined, or who will be intellectually gifted (quick, attentive, with a mind like a trap) "does not by itself imply," as Kamm writes,[87] that one would not care about a child who turned out differently—say a girl, or somehow disabled, or not all that interested in mathematics or music, or of ordinary intelligence, or for that matter "slow." But still, should expectations not be met, one might in fact be deeply disappointed *in the child*, and not only disappointed for him or her or that "resources" had been wasted.

As Schwartz has observed in his book *The Paradox of Choice*, the more choice we have, the higher our expectations tend to become, making us vulnerable to what he calls "the curse of discernment."[88] By contrast, both Kamm and Brock write as if parents never reject a child for failing to meet expectations, or that failure to accept and love one's child unconditionally is next to impossible given current child-rearing practices—as if abandonment and emotional estrangement, especially by fathers, were only remote theoretical possibilities.[89] Dismissing the relevance of the use of abortion when a fetus is discovered to be of the "wrong" sex or to have a genetic condition like Down or Turner's syndrome, Brock writes that "[f]ew if any parents would be prepared to kill an already born child because it developed a serious genetic disease or disability that had not been anticipated."[90] It is a lengthy leap, however, from this observation to the confident conclusion that few if any parents of a genetically enhanced child who did not meet expectations (and perhaps dearly bought expectations) would be disappointed *in* or *with* this child rather than only *for* him or her. The phenomenon of the "tentative pregnancy"—pregnancy pending the findings of prenatal diagnostic testing—suggests, not that the disappointed parent is likely to kill his or her born child (we may hope that Brock is right that far), but that parental acceptance of born children, like that of fetuses, cannot be taken for granted. Barbara Katz Rothman asks, "What does it do to motherhood, to women, and to men as fathers, too, when we make parental acceptance conditional, pending further testing?"[91] The mother whose acceptance is conditional might be interpreted as holding: "I have a choice of which child I'll have. Some of my possible children will likely have better lives than others. I want things to go as well as possible for whatever child I have."[92] Drawing on extensive interviews, Katz Rothman proposes, however, a more disturbing interpretation: "We ask the mother and her family to say, in essence, 'These are my standards. If you meet these standards of acceptability, then you are mine and I will love and accept you totally. After you pass this test.'"[93]

In this regard, we would do well to think about why parents might be drawn to genetic enhancement. Yes, it might simply be to "bring about something good" for a child, to use Kamm's language again; but can we not realistically imagine other, less rosy possibilities? Here Sandel's critique of the argument from precedent is relevant. As Sandel concedes, "improving children through genetic engineering is similar in spirit to the heavily managed, high-pressure child-rearing that is now common," at least in the circles most likely to embrace genetic technologies. "But this similarity," he goes on, "does not vindicate genetic enhancement. On the contrary, it highlights a problem with the trend toward hyperparenting,"[94] his word for the practice of pushing and "enriching" children toward ever greater heights, with the goal of positioning them to attain what are, from the parents' perspective, highly desirable social goods: the best schools, the best jobs, the best spouses—and the best (grand) children in turn. To repeat, yes, genetic enhancement might be sought simply to "bring about something good for the child"; but it seems strikingly naïve to fail to recognize that, within modern consumer cultures, the goods sought would often be, at bottom, parents' own, which might well make a significant difference for how parents would feel toward or "care about" a child, perhaps especially as he or she neared the identity-defining years of adolescence.

Whereas the so-called good enough parent identifies with his or her child and so adjusts his or her parenting for the child's own good according to his or her developing needs and interests,[95] it is not difficult to imagine a parent who had genetically enhanced his or her child demanding, as a condition of parental love, that the child conform to the parent's vision of the good. What is violated here is not so much the child's right to an open future as the parental obligation of love. Yes, such a parent could be criticized for failing to respect his or her child's autonomy, but it is the child's *present* autonomy, not the child's future autonomy, that the parent disregards. Accordingly, as Claudia Mills has observed, "[t]he wrong of overly directive child rearing" is then not only a sin against autonomy but "a sin against love" inasmuch as the parent "fails to accept and love the actual child here in front of us right now."[96] Interestingly, it is here that the Amish stand open to criticism. To put the point gently, if Amish parents have a failing, it looks to be a failing in love, inasmuch as it is made conditional on a child's electing to stay within the community.[97]

By way of conclusion, it must be acknowledged that this concern that I have raised is, of course, speculative, and more or less as Kant used this term: "Theoretical knowledge is speculative if it concerns an object . . . which cannot be reached in any experience."[98] Perhaps in the future we will have concrete data to discuss the ethics of prenatal genetic enhancement (in particular its effects on the parent-child relationship), but for now whatever we say cannot be confirmed empirically. Again in Kantian terms, for now whatever we say will then be "empty"—it will lack the fulfillment that only experience can bring—but it need not be "blind": even Kant allowed that "exercise[s] of the imagination in the company of reason" may provide insight so long as we can draw analogies between objects known to us (present-day "hyperparents") and the object of our speculation (parents who would be drawn to genetically enhancing children).[99] In any event, to rule out speculation here (say, to dismiss it as "mere speculation"[100]) is to run the risk that ethics will come too late.

It could be countered, of course, that to rule out prenatal genetic enhancement would be to succumb to speculative fear mongering about new technologies. To be clear, then, I do not pretend to have presented any so-called conclusive moral reasons against prenatal genetic enhancement.[101] In other words, I do not claim that it is always wrong for this or that reason, or that it cannot be morally permissible, praiseworthy, or perhaps even morally obligatory (as, for example, genetically enhancing a child's immune system might prove to be). But I think that the reasons to be wary of the practice of prenatal genetic enhancement extend well beyond the worry that some enhancements might violate a child's right to an open future. Would-be parents and genetic counselors also have reason to be wary of the practice of genetic enhancement, not because of the enhancements themselves, which in the abstract often appear unobjectionable, but in context, which is to say in view of how at least some enhancements might figure in, and potentially disfigure, parent-children relationships.[102]

A possible position is this: if genetic enhancements become available, some people will use them as part of their hyperparenting. Others will use the enhancements more judiciously. The problem is with the hyperparenting mentality and not with the enhancements themselves. Accordingly, we should work against the folly of hyperparenting and try to carve out a reasonable space for the use of genetic enhancements.[103] Similarly, Stephen Wilkinson has claimed that what is problematic is "not the *desire to select*" a child's characteristics, "but rather the *plan to reject* the child if it does not live up to expectations." Further, "it is entirely possible to want to select characteristics while not having this problematic attitude of rejection," just as it is possible to have the problematic attitude of rejection while *not* using any selection technologies.[104] (For this last possibility, Wilkinson gives the example of parents who do not sex select, yet are disposed to reject a child of "the 'wrong' sex."[105])

How could one disagree with this position? It is eminently reasonable. Wilkinson is surely right that what is problematic is the disposition to reject one's child if he or she does not please one better, and he is also surely right that there is no necessary, logical connection between using genetic enhancements (or other selection technologies) and falling afoul of what he terms the principle of unconditional parental love. But we should not deceive ourselves here. In Plato's heaven, the practice of genetic enhancement might present little reason to worry. Within modern consumer cultures, the prospect is surely different. Schwartz suggests that "a wide array of options can turn people into maximizers," which is to say people who "seek and accept only the best" and who are loathe to compromise with refractory realities.[106] If this is right, then decoupling the "hyperparenting mentality" and the enhancements themselves will prove easier said than done. Social science certainly gives us no reason to hold that parents who turn to genetic enhancements will necessarily, logically be disposed to reject their children should they not satisfy expectations. Should our powers of "choosing tomorrow's children"—the title of Wilkinson's book—be much increased, however, it does appear reasonable to think that expectations will escalate, and consequently parental distress as well when genetically enhanced children do not please their parents better. The main problem with choosing tomorrow's children may not be what it will do directly to these children. Instead, it appears that the problem to worry about is what it will do to these children's parents and thus to children indirectly.

6   Back from the Future
Paying for the Priceless Child

One of the most provocative, if not shocking, moments of Hugh LaFollette's proposal that prospective parents be licensed (referenced in passing toward the end of chapter 4) comes in his response to the objection that "we could never adequately, reasonably, and fairly enforce such a program" should persons go ahead and have children against its rules. LaFollette suggests that "[w]e might not punish parents at all—we might just remove the children and put them up for adoption."[1] What is shocking is the suggestion that losing one's child would not constitute a punishment: roughly, the deprivation of a good to which one would otherwise have a right (for example, freedom). The removal of one's child would not be a punishment, by LaFollette's lights, since one has only a conditional right to one's child to begin with: that is, a right conditional on somehow proving, in advance, that one would make a fit parent.[2]

LaFollette speculates that the root of opposition to his proposal is the belief that children belong to parents as a piece of property does.[3] After all, it might be claimed, parents do a bit of work—they quite literally mix themselves together—to produce the being in question. And on at least Locke's theory of property, it is by mixing our labor with things in nature that we make these things our own.[4] But I think it is more reasonable to suppose that the root of opposition is different. As I have already noted (likewise at the end of chapter 4), if the state had the power to prevent reproduction by ordinary means, there is little power that the state would not have. The state's power would encompass our bodies and extend over the most intimate domains of our formerly "private" lives. Further, LaFollette's proposal would put in the hands of the state the power to deprive one of what, for many persons, is a critical source of meaning and purpose in life: namely, a relationship with a child of one's own.[5] By calling a child one's own, one need not be claiming, of course, that the child belongs to one as a piece of property does, which one is largely free to use or abuse as one likes. Instead, to call one's child one's own, like calling one's spouse one's own, is typically to indicate a special, intimate relationship, and what's more a relationship that requires a significant measure of privacy and autonomy in order to be what it is. Invasive oversight and correction would likely transform the terms of the relationship. Just imagine a "nanny state" pecking at all of one's decisions. One's child might cease to feel one's own—just as one's parent might, should the security of the relationship constantly be threatened by the prospect of state intervention.[6]

The point of LaFollette's proposal, it must be acknowledged, is to protect children from the worst abuses of very bad parents.[7] And LaFollette does have a point that some parents can be very bad, such that we might wish they had never become parents at all. There are even grounds for thinking that LaFollette's proposal is not radical enough. As Francis Schrag has reflected, "Our families [may] provide us, when young, with the first glimmer of life in heaven"—but also "in hell."[8] Sadly, there is then a case to be made that it would be better to be born into a society with no families at all than to be born into the worst of families.

Throughout this book, I have extolled family, in the persons of parents, as an answer to life's loneliness and a justification for the mixed benefit of being brought into being. But if only every child were so fortunate. A possible response to my argument in this book is that it is all fine and well, but also too idealistic. More precisely, it might be wondered what bearing, if any, my so-called ideal theory has on this quite nonideal world of ours afflicted by poverty; rife with injustice; and populated not only by competent, loving parents with the means to do as they should, but abusive parents, sick parents, parents suffering from the spectrum of human ills and frailties—and children then suffering too.[9] Moreover, it might be objected that, apart from some critical comments in chapter 5 about "hyperparenting," I have had all too little to say against the tendency of parents, at least in so-called first-world countries like the United States, to "devote themselves to doing the best for *their own* children, rather than also to concern themselves with the needs of others, in particular, other children."[10] Readers might recall here my observation in the book's introduction that children have become a private luxury.

The aim of this closing chapter is to speak to the question of public responsibility for children. Laying out a full answer would take another and likely rather longer book, one more conversant in public policy and family law than I am prepared to offer. But it is important, in this context, to speak even briefly to the question, for philosophy nonetheless has a contribution to make here: namely, to consider whether there are reasons to think that current practices should be different in some basic way. To be clear, what I do in this chapter is no more than to *initiate* an analysis of public responsibility for children; no doubt this analysis could be deepened by considering at greater length the proper relationship between "man and state." My focus is more circumscribed.[11] I claim that, within the framework of a liberal state, public responsibility for children is not inconsiderable, *despite and even because of* the great value that we place on our own children. To make this case, it is helpful to consider another, even less "modest" proposal than LaFollette's: namely, that the family be abolished. I think that there is good reason to reject this proposal as well, but not without recognizing that this rejection comes with costs that call for compensation. (By the way, there is some literature on public responsibility and children, but it focuses on a society's obligations toward *parents*, not children, which is where I focus instead.[12])

§1. INJUSTICE AND THE FAMILY

As many readers will know, the status of the family in a just society has long been a source of uneasiness and contention among philosophers. Two great theorists of justice, one ancient and the other contemporary, can be cited in this regard: Plato and Rawls.

In the *Republic*, Plato's Socrates explains to Glaucon and Adeimantus—ironically, Plato's brothers—that all the guardians of his city-in-speech will see and treat one another as brother, sister, father, mother, son, or daughter.[13] The upshot is that no guardian effectively will have a family of his own, which is to say brothers, sisters, and so forth exclusive to him and not shared by all the other persons in his class. The goal is to ensure that the guardians use the phrase "my own" about the same things as much as possible. What Socrates fears is the prospect of the guardians' "draw[ing] the city apart by not all giving the name 'my own' to the same thing, but different men giving it to different things—one man dragging off to his own house whatever he can get his hands on apart from the others, another being separate in his own house with his separate women and children, introducing private pleasures and griefs"—and before long the spirit of faction, with each citizen out for himself and his family rather than concerned about the good of the whole.[14] Socrates goes so far as to say that the guardians would possess "nothing private but the body, while the rest is in common."[15] Read closely, the text may be taken as suggesting here that, inasmuch as the body resists "communization," Socrates's vision of a perfectly just city can never fully be realized: speech cannot pass to deed. The body poses an insuperable obstacle. The same objection, it should not be overlooked, applies to LaFollette's proposed regime. His suggestion that "[w]e might not punish parents at all—we might just remove the children" is implicit acknowledgment of the limits of state control. Whereas Plato, however, may be read as aware of the dangers of seeking to realize perfect justice, LaFollette's suggestion seems perfectly sincere.

One lesson that can be drawn from the *Republic* is that the family works against the realization of justice inasmuch as it breeds special interests among citizens. So it is today that, as I quoted Viviana Zelizer to observe in this book's introduction, while we place great value on children of our *own*, our society shows on the whole a "collective indifference to other people's children."[16] Of course, as we saw in chapter 5, there is sometimes lively interest in the subject of how other people's children are to be educated and raised. But, in the United States, this interest has not translated, by way of example, into fundamentally changing how we fund our public schools.

The tension if not conflict between justice and the family becomes yet more striking against the background of a commitment to equality of opportunity, also called equal life chances. Here Rawls's theory of justice can be called on for evidence. As is well known, Rawls articulates two principles of justice. The first is that "[e]ach person is to have an equal right to the most extensive total system of equal basic liberties compatible with a similar system of liberty for all." The second is that "[s]ocial and economic inequalities are to be arranged so that they are both (a) to the greatest benefit of the least advantaged," the so-called difference principle; "and (b) attached to offices and positions open to all under conditions of fair equality of opportunity."[17] Rawls specifies that, despite this order of presentation, "fair opportunity is prior to the difference principle," meaning that conditions of fair equality of opportunity must be satisfied before we go on to consider how to arrange inequalities to the greatest benefit of the least advantaged.[18] But there is a problem here, which Rawls himself acknowledges. In his own words, "the principle of fair opportunity can be only imperfectly carried out, at least as long as the institution of the family exists,"[19] acknowledgment of what one of his critics terms "the overwhelming effect of family background on life chances."[20]

In the end, Rawls does not solve this problem. "Is the family to be abolished then?" he asks toward the conclusion of his book. "Taken by itself and given a certain primacy, the idea of equal opportunity inclines in this direction. But within the context of the theory of justice as a whole, there is much less urgency to take this course,"[21] a claim that he supports by invoking the difference principle:

> The acknowledgement of the difference principle redefines the grounds for social inequalities as conceived in the system of liberal equality. . . . We are more ready to dwell on our good fortune now that these differences are made to work to our advantage, rather than be downcast by how much better off we might have been had we had an equal chance along with others if only all social barriers had been removed.[22]

The reason why this argumentative move does not work is that it violates or at the very least relaxes Rawls's own specification that "fair opportunity is prior to the difference principle," an ordering that he was at pains to establish lest we have to fall back on intuition in balancing principles.[23] As Schrag has noted, "there seems to be no basis within Rawls's system for excepting the family from the stringencies imposed" by his ordering of the principles. Given that Rawls does not present the family as a primary good that all parties would choose in the original position, it seems that, again in Schrag's words, "Rawls's retention of the nuclear family structure reflects . . . an unwillingness on his part to accept all of the implications of his own theory."[24]

The problem here is not, moreover, unique to Rawls's theory. James Fishkin has argued that "[o]nce the role of the family is accounted for, the conflict between liberty and equality becomes an unavoidable problem at the core of liberal theory."[25] Fishkin calls attention in this regard to what he terms a "trilemma": to change the image a bit, how to square commitment to equality of life chances, autonomy of the family, and a so-called principle of merit, the last of which ensures fairness in the evaluation of qualifications for positions (more precisely, that positions be assigned on the basis of skills, credentials, and motivation). Commitment to any two of these three requires sacrificing the third. By way of example, there is no way to keep in place the autonomy of the family and yet to equalize life chances without sacrificing the principle of merit: "Only a process of assignment that was applied regardless of meritocratic factors could equalize life chances despite differential talent development."[26] Should we be unwilling to sacrifice the principle of merit yet seek still to equalize life chances, it appears that only a system of collective or communal child rearing, say on the model of the Israeli *kibbutz*, would prove effective. For "anything short of such a large-scale alternative would probably provide only an imperfect barrier between the inequalities of the parental generation and the developmental processes affecting its children."[27]

Given a choice among child-rearing structures, it could well be, as Schrag proposes, that "a rational person in the original position following a [so-called] maximin strategy"—that is, adopting that alternative the worst outcome of which is superior to the worst outcomes of the others—"would choose the communal structure."[28] After all, within it "the resources (material, intellectual, psychological) of the *entire* community are made available to *every* child as opposed to the familial arrangement wherein the child's opportunities depend to a large extent on the resources the family he is born into happen to possess."[29] But this choice, however rational and compelling when we consider how bad the worst of families can be, seems wrong. That is, the choice to abolish the family cuts against our aspiration for the good, which in this case is stronger than our aversion to the bad—as Rawls's retention of the family, despite his theoretical commitments, appears to attest. In this light, the conclusion seems warranted that, though justice may be, as Rawls claims, "the first virtue of social institutions,"[30] it is not the first virtue of all human associations.[31] The family as we know it embodies value that ought not to be sacrificed even to the demands of justice.

What is valuable about the family, I think, is its nurturance of (or at least potential to nurture) deep, intimate relationships of a kind that it appears cannot readily be had elsewhere. Schrag reaches for Martin Buber's concept of the I-You relationship in order to explain what is at stake here. The love in an I-You relationship "clings to a unique individual, not to a set of properties," and accordingly is not transferrable to someone else who might happen to have the same properties and perhaps more or better.[32] Instead, the persons in an I-You relationship encounter one another, as it were, "without properties," and stand committed to one another unconditionally. In chapter 1, I spoke similarly of relationships that can be counted on *as* given, based not on the features of the beloved, but more simply, and even mysteriously, on that person's *being*. The mystery here should not be downplayed or dismissed. That we can have relationships of unconditional love with one another—broken and flawed as we human beings are—is a thing worthy of wonder. Now, it may well be that there are relationships of unconditional love other than family relationships, but these seem rarer, and it is significant that they are often described as *like* family relationships: someone is said to be "like a sister," or "like a brother," etc.—lending credence to the claim that the family has the potential to foster relationships of a special kind. As Schrag puts this claim, "The situation in which a father and a mother have sole and total responsibility for the rearing of their child is one which fosters the exclusiveness, the sense of individual uniqueness which characterizes the I-You encounter."[33] To demand that we sacrifice such relationships in the name of justice is surely to ask too much.

§2. MAKING GOOD

What, then, are we to do? A possible response, of course, is simply to dismiss the demands of justice, or in any event (allowing for different theories of justice from Rawls's) to renounce our commitment to equality of opportunity. But this response seems too easy, and false to the dilemma at hand. The claim that commitment to equal opportunity conflicts with commitment to the institution of the family represents, I think, an instance of what Niko Kolodny calls the "more general truth that not everything of value can be realized within a single social formation."[34] More fully, there are two "ought's" at work here, corresponding to two values that each call for realization. On the one hand, we ought to preserve the family given the relationships that it nurtures. On the other hand, we ought to give all children roughly equal chances in life, for every child deserves a "level playing field," so to speak, from which to make his or her start. But differences in familial resources—intellectual, psychological, and spiritual as well as material—mean that children enter life with vastly different life chances. The playing field is tilted from the

start. Leveling down differences might be possible over several genera-
tions, but at the cost of sacrificing the principle of merit in favor of a
policy of reverse discrimination, assigning positions on a basis other than
skills, credentials, and motivation.[35] By contrast, strategies of leveling-
up appear more attractive, but also inadequate. Improving nutrition,
health care, and preschool education for the worst off would not suffice
to equalize developmental conditions.[36] As Fishkin puts the point here,
even under ideal conditions, our commitments "cannot all be realized
simultaneously." He concludes that "[w]e must either abandon one or
more of these commitments, or we must modify them by admitting their
susceptibility to sacrifice" and compromise. Otherwise we put forth "an
incoherent ideal for public policy"—an accusation that he directs against
Rawls.[37]

The question to consider is whether there is some way to honor our
commitment to equal opportunity—which I take to be essential to a liberal state, or indeed to any community committed to a robust common
good—while yet prioritizing our commitment to the family. They conflict,
but need this be the final word? Faced with a conflict between beliefs, we
typically seek to determine which belief is stronger. The other belief is
then either revised, weakened, or abandoned.[38] Conflict between moral
convictions, like conflict between desires, is often different. Here, too, we
typically seek to determine which obligation is stronger—yet without any
necessity or even pressure to conclude that the other obligation must be
false and so discarded.[39] The obligation that we decide against need not
even be weakened in our estimation. To the contrary, we might consider
ourselves to have strong reasons to pursue it, but just not as strong as
the reasons to pursue the obligation that we have prioritized.[40] Now, in
some cases, after we have had to decide for one obligation over another,
the only way that we have to acknowledge the resulting loss of value is to
feel and express regret. We regret that circumstances were such that we
could not have done differently—that it was not possible for us to realize
both of the values in question. In other cases, however, it is open to us to
take some measures to try to make up for the value lost—though it is clear
that the best we can do is to try to make good after having been unable
to do entirely right.

The conflict between commitment to equal opportunity and commitment to the institution of the family is the latter sort of case: it leaves us
with means of redress other than regret; there are ways to try to make
up for, though not entirely to recuperate, what is lost when we prioritize
the family despite the significant inequalities that it produces. By way
of example, we might invest significantly in improving nutrition, health
care, and preschool education for the worst off. Though, as I have noted,
these measures would not suffice to realize the ideal of equal life chances,
they would bring real-life benefits to many and so give children much
better chances in life than they would otherwise have.[41]

An objection to anticipate here is that it is artificial to speak of choosing to prioritize the family over equal life chances. How many among us, in cherishing and giving special treatment to *our own* (children, parents, siblings), do so after deliberation over whether commitment to the institution of the family ought to take priority over commitment to equal life chances? Instead, we live in a society where, in Rawls's matter-of-fact language, "the institution of the family exists" and so "the principle of fair opportunity can be only imperfectly carried out," irrespective of whatever dictates hypothetical decision procedures like the original position might yield. Yet part of the value of hypothetical decision procedures is precisely to remind us that ways of life that we take for granted do not come without costs, or in other words that these ways of life are not value free: they reflect priorities and so, in a sense, choices that have been made for us, whether after deliberation or not. Moreover, hypothetical decision procedures, like the original position, give us the opportunity to decide whether these priorities ought, on reflection, to be endorsed. If so, they become our choices after all, for which we then assume responsibility.

Here is the upshot. If we are unwilling to conclude that, in the name of equal life chances for all children, the family ought to be abolished in favor of some structure of communal child rearing—as I believe we have good reason to be unwilling to conclude—then we, as a liberal political society committed to equal opportunity, have a duty to *compensate* children who suffer deprivation from this choice of ours. In other words, if we decide that the value of having *our own* children (Zelizer's "the priceless child") is greater than the value of seeking to assure all children equal life chances, then we owe it to children in need to take measures to assure that they have at least *good* life chances, though there is no pretending that these will be the equal of children with better fortunes in life.

To repeat from the beginning of this discussion, laying out a full answer to the question of public responsibility for children would take another and likely rather longer book, and what's more one going beyond the competence of at least this philosopher. A full answer would have to bear concretely on such matters as taxation, the funding of public education, health care, child support, and institutional and foster care (including responsibilities toward so-called emancipated foster youth, which is to say youth who have aged out of the system).[42] Social scientists, social workers, legal scholars, and legislators all have parts to play here; so too do historians, who can teach us about how "welfare as we know it" came to be in the United States and throw light on the perils to children of rolling back such developments as Aid to Dependent Children (ended in 1996 under the name Aid to Families with Dependent Children).[43] What falls to philosophy is to indicate the grounds and dimensions of our responsibility, not to lay out institutional solutions.

A philosophical argument like my own does, however, yield some constructive conclusions. One implication of my argument about public responsibility for children is that individual citizens of liberal democracies have a duty to support institutional reforms toward improving the lives of children in need. That much seems clear and relatively simple, though of course one must then be well informed about both the lot of children in our society and realistic ways forward.[44] A second implication hits closer to home. This is that there is a duty for individuals to do what *they* can for children in need, in recognition that better government is not the answer to all problems. The duty in question here is a so-called imperfect duty inasmuch as how, when, and to whom it is to be discharged fall to discretion. What is obligatory is to make it one's policy, so to speak, to help children who suffer deprivation because of the great value we place on having children of *our own*—that is, to help children whose lives might well be better if children were reared in common, with all the resources of the community brought to bear, rather than in the setting of the family. To give some concrete examples of how this duty might be discharged, one might, at some point in one's life, serve as a foster parent, participate in Big Brothers Big Sisters, give money to charities that work with and for children, or volunteer or even teach in an inner-city school. And one should certainly seek to be sensitive to, and to correct, excessive spending on one's own.[45] The goal, in all these cases, would be the same: while not eliminating special concern for one's own, to widen the circle of one's concern in the name of greater justice. Other people's children, I submit, deserve as much.

Notes

NOTES TO THE INTRODUCTION

1. The case is that of Sharon Duchesneau and Candy McCullough. See, for example, Michael Parker, "An Ordinary Chance of a Desirable Existence," in *Procreation and Parenthood: The Ethics of Bearing and Rearing Children*, eds. David Archard and David Benatar (Oxford: Oxford University Press, 2010), 57–77, at 62–64.
2. See, for example, Dena S. Davis, "Genetic Dilemmas and the Child's Right to an Open Future," *Hastings Center Report* 27/2 (1997): 7–15; and Jonathan Glover, *Choosing Children: Genes, Disability, and Design* (Oxford: Oxford University Press, 2006), 5 and 63–72.
3. See Bruno Bettelheim, *A Good Enough Parent: A Book on Child-Rearing* (New York: Alfred A. Knopf, 1987), the title of which is derived, as Bettelheim acknowledges, "from D. W. Winnicott's concept of the 'good enough' mother" (ix), developed in particular in Winnicott's *The Maturational Processes and the Facilitating Environment: Studies in the Theory of Emotional Development* (New York: International Universities Press, 1965). What is perhaps most distinctive to the good enough mother, as Winnicott uses the term, is her identification with the infant (71, 147) and so "high degree of adaption . . . to the infant's needs" (96, 148). As he writes, "One could use the word 'love' here, at the risk of sounding sentimental" (72).
4. Onora O'Neill, "Children's Rights and Children's Lives," *Ethics* 98 (1988): 445–463, at 445.
5. See Colin Heydt, "Practical Ethics in Eighteenth-Century Britain," in *The Oxford Handbook of Eighteenth-Century British Philosophy*, ed. James Harris (Oxford: Oxford University Press, 2013), 369–389. For the British moralists of this era, so-called private rights, the rights that we have as human beings, break down into perfect rights, "claims of *justice*" that we can make against others; and imperfect rights, "claims of *humanity* that we have against one another" toward, for example, benevolence and positive assistance, pity, gratitude, and forgiveness (382). Not only can the fulfillment of imperfect rights usually not be demanded or compelled; just what actions would fulfill these rights usually can be specified only vaguely and indeterminately. As Heydt puts this point, "In other words, how much gratitude I deserve from you is vague is a way that what I owe to another to fulfill a contract is not" (382).
6. O'Neill, "The 'Good Enough' Parent in the Age of the New Reproductive Technologies," in *The Ethics of Genetics in Human Procreation*, eds. Hille Haker and Deryck Beyleveld (Aldershot: Ashgate, 2000), 33–48, at 37.

7. Mary Shelley, *Frankenstein*, ed. J. Paul Hunter (New York: W. W. Norton, 1996), 67; see also 151. The creature comes to life "on a dreary night of November" (see 34); Victor Frankenstein first feels the duties of a creator in August of the next year (67).

8. Somewhat like God in Genesis 2, Victor bypasses the natural order in making, rather than begetting, his creature, born not from a relationship with a woman but by his own "painful labour" in natural philosophy, until at last he discovered "the cause of generation and life" and became "capable of bestowing animation upon lifeless matter" (ibid., 30–31). Yet, unlike God in Genesis 2, Victor is both constrained by the matter that he has to work with—detritus from "the dissecting room and the slaughter house"—and pressed by time, such that, "contrary to [his] first intention," he decides in the end "to make the being of gigantic stature; that is to say, about eight-feet in height, and proportionably large" (31–32). When at last he "infuse[s] a spark of being into the lifeless thing" in his laboratory, the creature who comes to life not only, then, is of superhuman size, but bears the canker of death in its flesh (34). The creature accordingly provokes in Victor "breathless horror and disgust," and Victor's first reaction to him is to rush out of the room (34). Seeking "a few moments of forgetfulness," Victor falls asleep, only to be "disturbed by the wildest dreams" in which the woman he is destined to marry, on receiving a kiss from his lips, turns in his arms into the corpse of his dead mother (34). We are to understand, it seems, that "Mother Nature" does not take well to her violation. At that moment, Victor wakes to behold, in his words, "the wretch—the miserable monster whom I had created. . . . His jaws opened, and he muttered some inarticulate sounds, while a grin wrinkled his cheeks. He might have spoken, but I did not hear; one hand was stretched out, seemingly to detain me, but I escaped," rushing now out of the house, forever abandoning the creature to his own devices (35). By contrast, God had prepared a garden for the work of his hands.

9. See Samuel Scheffler's "non-reductionist" account of special responsibilities in his "Relationships and Responsibilities," *Philosophy and Public Affairs* 26 (1997): 189–209.

10. Ordinary language makes it difficult to observe the distinction between permissibility (nothing stands, morally, in the way of a course of action) and justification (there is positive moral reason to do the action in question). For example, we say that an action that is impermissible cannot be justified. But I ask readers to keep the distinction in mind.

11. Should a reader be interested in my position, however, see my article "A Riskier Discourse," *Commonweal*, November 23, 2012, 16–20.

12. Rivka Weinberg, "The Moral Complexity of Sperm Donation," *Bioethics* 22 (2008): 166–178, at 168, 169.

13. Elizabeth Brake, "Fatherhood and Child Support: Do Men Have a Right to Choose?" *Journal of Applied Philosophy* 22 (2005): 55–73, at 68.

14. Viviana A. Zelizer, *Pricing the Priceless Child: The Changing Social Value of Children* (Princeton, NJ: Princeton University Press, 1994), 170, 195.

15. Anne L. Alstott, *No Exit: What Parents Owe Their Children and What Society Owes Parents* (Oxford: Oxford University Press, 2004), 50.

16. Zelizer, *Pricing the Priceless Child*, xiii.

17. Ibid., 216.

18. Drew D. Hansen, "The American Invention of Child Support: Dependency and Punishment in Early American Child Support Law," *Yale Law Journal* 108 (1999): 1123–1153, at 1124. As Hansen observes, "the modern child support system [in the United States] is centrally concerned with saving

public money," to the detriment of children whose noncustodial fathers lack economic means. See 1151, 1152.

NOTES TO CHAPTER 1

1. John Milton, *Paradise Lost*, in *The Complete Poetical Works of John Milton* (New York: Thomas Y. Crowell, 1892), bk. 10, lines 743–745, p. 236.
2. Friedrich Nietzsche, *Die Geburt der Tragödie* (Stuttgart: Philipp Reclam, 1993), ch. 3, p. 29; *The Birth of Tragedy*, trans. Walter Kaufmann (New York: Random House, 1967), 42.
3. Job 3:3–5 (NRSV).
4. Philip Larkin, "This Be The Verse," in *Collected Poems*, ed. Anthony Thwaite (New York: Farrar, Straus and Giroux, 2003), 142. The poem's first line (easily googled) is famous for its vulgarity.
5. The poem here concurs, interestingly, with the judgment of Adam contemplating the human condition after the fall, namely, bound by sin passed from generation to generation. "'But this will not serve/,'" Adam says: "'All that I . . . shall beget/ Is propagated curse.'" See *Paradise Lost*, bk. 10, lines 727–729, p. 236.
6. But see David Benatar, "Why It Is Better Never to Come into Existence," *American Philosophical Quarterly* 34 (1997): 345–355, developed at length in *Better Never to Have Been: The Harm of Coming into Existence* (Oxford: Oxford University Press, 2006). See also, however, extensive criticisms of the argument in Elizabeth Harman "Critical Study," *Noûs* 43 (2009): 776–785; David Boonin, "Better to Be," *South African Journal of Philosophy* 31 (2012): 10–25; and Rivka Weinberg, "Is Having Children Always Wrong?" *South African Journal of Philosophy* 31 (2012): 26–37. I share these critics' rejection of Benatar's basic argument.
7. For analyses of "wrongful life" that avoid the logical pitfalls surrounding this concept, see Jeff McMahan, "Wrongful Life: Paradoxes in the Morality of Causing People to Exist," in *Rational Commitment and Social Justice: Essays for Gregory Kavka*, eds. Jules L. Coleman and Christopher W. Morris (Cambridge: Cambridge University Press, 1998), 208–247, at 215; and Allen Buchanan, Dan W. Brock, Norman Daniels, and Daniel Wikler, *From Chance to Choice: Genetics and Justice* (Cambridge: Cambridge University Press, 2000), 234–235.
8. Derek Parfit, *Reasons and Persons* (Oxford: Oxford University Press, 1984), 378. For defense of this supposition, see Parfit, *Reasons and Persons*, 351–355; and McMahan, "Wrongful Life," 208–209.
9. Compare the Yiddish joke quoted by Robert Nozick in his *Anarchy, State, and Utopia* (New York: Basic Books, 1974), 337, n. 8: "—'Life is so terrible; it would be better never to have been conceived.'—'Yes, but who is so fortunate? Not one in a thousand.'"
10. John Harris, *Enhancing Evolution: The Ethical Case for Making Better People* (Princeton, NJ: Princeton University Press, 2007), 159. Compare John A. Robertson, *Children of Choice: Freedom and the New Reproductive Technologies* (Princeton, NJ: Princeton University Press, 1994), 122, on artificial insemination by donor and surrogacy, and then 169, on cloning.
11. By the way, Harris speaks of the "'non-identity' argument," not "problem" as Parfit called it. See Harris, *Enhancing Evolution*, 153.
12. I thank a referee for this analogy.
13. For a further engagement should the reader not be satisfied with this move, see Rivka Weinberg, "Identifying and Dissolving the Non-Identity

Problem," *Philosophical Studies* 137 (2008): 3–18. An important question is whether attempts at circumventing the non-identity problem, focusing on responsibilities "concerning the having of children," suffice to ground the claim that parents may do wrong even when no child has been harmed. Weinberg objects that attempts to bypass the problem of identifying who is harmed by procreative decisions fail to undermine the principle that "procreation is morally permissible so long as the future person's life is likely to be worth living" (5). Her own proposed solution turns on the claim that "existence . . . is something that all future people will have" and so should not "be taken as a gift we bestow which outweighs other burdens," which is how she claims existence is conceived by Parfit (16).

14. Glover, *Choosing Children*, 24. Compare Mary Warnock, "'The Good of the Child,'" *Bioethics* 1 (1987): 141–155, at 143–144.

15. See Alan Donagan, *The Theory of Morality* (Chicago: The University of Chicago Press, 1977), 101.

16. See John Boswell, *The Kindness of Strangers: The Abandonment of Children in Western Europe from Late Antiquity through the Renaissance* (New York: Pantheon, 1988), 24–25 on the extension of the word 'abandonment,' and 138–179 on the development of the moral tradition.

17. Donagan, *The Theory of Morality*, 101.

18. Ibid., 102.

19. For the concept of prima facie duty, see David Ross, *The Right and the Good*, ed. Philip Stratton-Lake (Oxford: Oxford University Press, 2002), 19–20, 28. For helpful clarifications, see the editor's introduction, xxxiii–xxxviii.

20. Michael J. Broyde, "Adoption, Personal Status, and Jewish Law," in *The Morality of Adoption: Socio-Psychological, Theological, and Legal Perspectives*, ed. Timothy P. Jackson (Grand Rapids, MI: Eerdmans, 2005), 128–147, at 129.

21. General Court of Massachusetts, "An Act to Provide for the Adoption of Children (1851)," in *Families by Law: An Adoption Reader*, eds. Naomi R. Cahn and Joan Heifetz Hollinger (New York: New York University Press, 2004), 9–10. See further Stephen B. Presser, "The Historical Background of the American Law of Adoption," *Journal of Family Law* 11 (1972): 443–516, especially 465–470.

22. It should finally be noted that the repudiation of full legal adoption does not necessarily entail the denigration of rearing children birthed by others. After all, the Hebrew prophets again and again enjoin care for the orphan. In Jewish thought, becoming "custodial parents" is a highly significant act, as it is "predicated on voluntary choice, which is the hallmark of all sacred covenantal relationships." See Broyde, "Adoption, Personal Status, and Jewish Law," 147. In Islam, the question appears to be more complicated. Like the prophets in the Hebrew Bible, the Qur'an enjoins care for orphans. Yet, as in Judaism, full legal adoption is prohibited, in Islam "by the *Shari'a* on the grounds of the Koran 33.4–5." See Dariusch Atighetchi, *Islamic Bioethics: Problems and Perspectives* (Dordrecht: Springer, 2007), 139. So-called testamentary adoption is not traditionally prohibited, yet in some Islamic countries it is understood to be. See, in this regard, Lydia Polgreen, "Overcoming Customs and Stigma, Sudan Gives Orphans a Lifeline," *New York Times*, April 5, 2008, section A.

23. See Mary B. Mahowald, "Relinquishment and Adoption: Are They Genuine Options?" *Cambridge Quarterly of Healthcare Ethics* 5 (1996): 437–439, at 439, noting the reaction of health-care workers to the decision of a

married woman, with three children at home, to give up for adoption a fourth child, born of an unwanted pregnancy after the woman had returned to the workforce.

24. Elizabeth Bartholet, *Family Bonds: Adoption and the Politics of Parenting* (Boston: Houghton Mifflin, 1993), 181. By the way, it is worth noting that the traditional position that adoption can be justified only *in extremis* might work against the pleas of advocates of traditional morality that pregnant women consider adoption in place of abortion. On this point, see Mahowald, "Relinquishment and Adoption," at 438–439.

25. Mary L. Shanley, "Fathers' Rights, Mothers' Wrongs? Reflections on Unwed Fathers' Rights and Sex Equality," *Hypatia* 10 (1995): 74–103, at 92.

26. Consider in this regard the controversy in the European Union over the use of "baby boxes," the modern analogue of the medieval foundling wheel. See (or listen to) Philip Reeves, "Spread of 'Baby Boxes' Alarms Europeans," National Public Radio, February 18, 2013, www.npr.org/2013/02/18/172336348/spread-of-baby-boxes-alarms-europeans.

27. See John Robertson's "Surrogate Mothers: Not So Novel After All," *Hastings Center Report* 13/5 (1983): 28–34, which presents surrogacy as no different from adoption. Robertson claims that, as the practice of adoption already separates biological and social parenting and is seen as passing moral muster, surrogacy, which likewise separates biological and social parenting, should likewise be seen as passing moral muster. What this argument from precedent blatantly (and willfully?) ignores is that, in adoption, the child already exists and the separation of biological and social parenting is tolerated in the child's interests; in surrogacy, the separation of biological and social parenting is planned in advance of the child's conception.

28. Paul Lauritzen, *Pursuing Parenthood: Ethical Issues in Assisted Reproduction* (Bloomington: Indiana University Press, 1993), 128. See his chapter 6, "The Myth and Reality of Current Adoption Practice," 119–134.

29. Boswell, *The Kindness of Strangers*, 136, 264, 328.

30. The Baby M case is the prime exhibit. See for two quite different takes Lori B. Andrews, "Surrogate Motherhood: The Challenge for Feminists," *Journal of Law, Medicine, and Health Care* 16 (1988): 72–80; and Katha Pollitt, "The Strange Case of Baby M," *The Nation*, May 23, 1987, www.thenation.com/article/strange-case-baby-m.

31. Leon R. Kass, "The Meaning of Life—in the Laboratory," in *Life, Liberty and the Defense of Dignity: The Challenge for Bioethics* (San Francisco: Encounter, 2002), 81–117, at 98. Compare Edgar Page, "Donation, Surrogacy and Adoption," *Journal of Applied Philosophy* 2 (1985): 161–167, at 167; and Herbert T. Krimmel, "The Case against Surrogate Parenting," *Hastings Center Report* 13/5 (1983): 35–39, at 36–37.

32. I take Kass's reasoning to be that encouraging people to generate children for others to adopt would lead to baby markets because these children would be generated not as ends in themselves but as mere means to another purpose, namely, adoption by others. Once children are reduced to mere means, then they can logically be used for other purposes too, like profit making in baby markets.

33. Kass, "The Meaning of Life—in the Laboratory," in *Life, Liberty and the Defense of Dignity*, 98, 100. Compare in this regard article 8 of the United Nations Convention on the Rights of the Child, which speaks of "the right of the child to preserve his or her identity" (§1). See www2.ohchr.org/english/law/crc.htm.

34. Krimmel, "Surrogate Mother Arrangements from the Perspective of the Child," *Logos* 9 (1988): 97–112, at 98.

35. Immanuel Kant, *Grundlegung zur Metaphysik der Sitten*, ed. Karl Vorländer, 3rd ed. (Hamburg: Felix Meiner, 1965), 4:429, p. 52; *Groundwork of the Metaphysics of Morals*, trans. Mary Gregor (Cambridge: Cambridge University Press, 1997), 38.

36. Onora O'Neill, "Ending World Hunger," in *Matters of Life and Death: New Introductory Essays in Moral Philosophy*, ed. Tom Regan, 3rd ed. (New York: McGraw-Hill, 1993), 235–279, at 261. See also Christine Korsgaard, "The Right to Lie: Kant on Dealing with Evil," in *Creating the Kingdom of Ends* (Cambridge: Cambridge University Press, 1996), 138. To put the point a bit differently, we have reason to be sure that the policy of our action (maxim) can be adopted by all (as a policy to lie, steal, or cheat off others could not be) because we have reason to respect persons. A policy that could not be adopted by all would be a policy that treats others as mere means to our own ends, rather than as ends in themselves (persons whose good and autonomy ought to be honored). It would be a policy parasitic on other persons.

37. Virginia Held, "Noncontractual Society: The Postpatriarchal Family as Model," in *Feminist Morality: Transforming Culture, Society, and Politics* (Chicago: The University of Chicago Press, 1993), 192–214, at 195 and 204.

38. See for discussion T. M. Scanlon, *Moral Dimensions: Permissibility, Meaning, Blame* (Cambridge, MA: Harvard University Press, 2008), 91–92.

39. See for an excellent literary example Philip Roth's *The Human Stain* (New York: Random House, 2000), 175–177. It matters deeply to Coleman Silk's son Markie to know his origins; it seems to matter less, if at all, to Coleman's several other children.

40. A. Phillips Griffiths, "Child Adoption and Identity," in *Philosophy and Practice*, ed. A. Phillips Griffiths (Cambridge: Cambridge University Press, 1985), 275–285, at 277.

41. Betty Jean Lifton, "Shared Identity Issues for Adoptees," in *Clinical and Practical Issues in Adoption: Bridging the Gap between Adoptees Placed as Infants and as Older Children*, eds. Victor Groza and Karen F. Rosenberg (Westport, CT: Praeger, 1998), 37–48, at 37 (italics mine). Lifton refers to Erikson's *Identity: Youth and Crisis* (New York: W. W. Norton, 1968).

42. Positive identity is characterized as "'a sense of psychological well-being, a feeling of being at home in one's body, of knowing where one is going, [and] an inner assuredness of anticipated recognition from those who count.'" See John Triseliotis, "Identity Formation and the Adopted Person Revisited," in *The Dynamics of Adoption: Social and Personal Perspectives*, eds. Amal Treacher and Ilan Katz (London: Jessica Kingsley, 2000), 81–97, at 89, who paraphrases Erikson's *Identity: Youth and Crisis*, 165.

43. Lifton, "Shared Identity Issues for Adoptees," 37.

44. Katarina Wegar, *Adoption, Identity, and Kinship: The Debate over Sealed Birth Records* (New Haven, CT: Yale University Press, 1997), x. Note the title of Lifton's paper: "*Shared* Identity Issues for Adoptees" (emphasis added). See also, for similar criticism to Wegar's, Mark A. Nolan and Diana M. Grace, "Should Adopted Children Be Granted Access to the Identity of Their Birth Parents? A Psychological Perspective," *Journal of Information Ethics* 12 (2003): 67–79, at 70–71.

45. See Wegar, *Adoption, Identity, and Kinship*, 115, for a striking example.

46. See, for a nice discussion, Jean Bethke Elshtain, "The Chosen Family," *The New Republic*, September 14 and 21, 1998, 45–54, at 52–54. See also Wegar, *Adoption, Identity, and Kinship*, 2, 45, 52, 76, 123, 131. To quote

only this last page, search activists "have emphasized the biological determinants of feelings of kinship and characterized the need to search as a genetic and universal biological imperative."

47. Sarah-Vaughan Brakman and Sally J. Scholz, "Adoption, ART, and a Re-Conception of the Maternal Body: Toward Embodied Maternity," *Hypatia* 21 (2006): 54–73, at 61. In this regard, it is illuminating to note that it is simply false that all adopted persons find it necessary to set out on "the search" in order to come to "confidence in . . . inner continuity amid change," though nowadays, due to changing family and social expectations, "the pressure is on those who do not search to do so." See for this point Triseliotis, "Identity Formation and the Adopted Person Revisited," 81. See also Gretchen Miller Wrobel, Harold D. Grotevant, and Ruth G. McRoy, "Adolescent Search for Birthparents: Who Moves Forward?" *Journal of Adolescent Research* 19 (2004): 132–151, at 133–134, 148.

48. Brakman and Scholz, "Adoption, ART, and a Re-Conception of the Maternal Body," 62.

49. See again Roth's *The Human Stain*, 175–177.

50. See Brakman and Scholz, "Adoption, ART, and a Re-Conception of the Maternal Body," 62.

51. Wrobel, Grotevant, and McRoy, "Adolescent Search for Birthparents," 136.

52. I thank Lydia Moland for this suggestion.

53. See Boswell, *The Kindness of Strangers*, 122, 127.

54. O'Neill, "The 'Good Enough' Parent in the Age of the New Reproductive Technologies," 41.

55. I owe the formulation of this contrast to Chelsea Gaudet. Compare Marilyn Friedman, *What Are Friends For? Feminist Perspectives on Personal Relationships and Moral Theory* (Ithaca, NY: Cornell University Press, 1993), 209: "friendship is a kind of achievement. Those who would be friends must exert themselves actively to sustain their relationship."

56. O'Neill, "The 'Good Enough' Parent in the Age of the New Reproductive Technologies," 41. For social-scientific support of these claims, see Triseliotis, "Identity Formation and the Adopted Person Revisited," 88–89; and David M. Brodzinsky, "A Stress and Coping Model of Adoption Adjustment," in *The Psychology of Adoption*, eds. David M. Brodzinsky and Marshall M. Schechter (New York: Oxford University Press, 1990), 3–24, at 7. Brodzinsky reports that "adopted children, once they come to realize the implications of being adopted, not only experience a loss of their biological parents and origins, but also [experience] a loss of stability in the relationship to their adoptive parents." So one reason why it would be "better *not* to have been chosen, but given," is that it is better to grow up without any question that the parent-child relationship might be conditional, or that it might (once more) be broken.

57. See also James Lindemann Nelson, "Genetic Narratives: Biology, Stories, and the Definition of the Family," *Health Matrix* 2 (1992): 71–83, especially 81: "the role of genetic connections in our lives can be seen, not as 'gene calling to gene,' but rather as a part of our interest in perceiving the connections between our lives and the lives of others—connections which add depth and richness to the continuing story in which we participate, and which can therefore be referred to as narrative connections."

58. Claudia Mills, "Duties to Aging Parents," in *Care of the Aged*, eds. James M. Humber and Robert F. Almeder (Totawa, NJ: Humana Press, 2003), 147–166, at 149.

59. Joseph Kupfer, "Can Parents and Children Be Friends?," *American Philosophical Quarterly* 27 (1990): 15–26, at 21.

60. Ibid., 22.
61. Ibid., 23. Arguably, unconditional love should not even be the ideal between romantic partners. See for this claim Derek Edyvane, "Against Unconditional Love," *Journal of Applied Philosophy* 20 (2003): 59–75.
62. See Stephen Wilkinson, *Choosing Tomorrow's Children: The Ethics of Selective Reproduction* (Oxford: Oxford University Press, 2010), 23.
63. O'Neill, "The 'Good Enough' Parent in the Age of the New Reproductive Technologies," 38.
64. See on this important point Bettelheim, *A Good Enough Parent*, 71 (on the child's great fear of abandonment), 296–297 (on the role of parental love in developing a child's "convictions about his own value as a person"), and 333 (on the role of parental love in giving a child "inner security").
65. Triseliotis, "Identity Formation and the Adopted Person Revisited," 88.
66. Of course, it is open to controversy which facts or offenses should count as serious enough to justify putting the relationship on hold. See on this point Wilkinson, *Choosing Tomorrow's Children*, 27.
67. See for documentation S. Matthew Liao, "The Right of Children to Be Loved," *The Journal of Political Philosophy* 14 (2006): 420–440, at 423–424. As Liao summarizes studies of children in institutions, "children who did not receive love but only adequate care became ill more frequently; their learning capacities deteriorated significantly; they became decreasingly interested in their environment; they failed to thrive physically by failing to gain height or weight or both; they suffered insomnia; they were constantly depressed; and they eventually developed severe learning disabilities" (423).
68. Simon Keller, *The Limits of Loyalty* (Cambridge: Cambridge University Press, 2007), 124. Compare, drawing from the Confucian tradition, Philip J. Ivanhoe, "Filial Piety as a Virtue," in *Working Virtue: Virtue Ethics and Contemporary Moral Problems*, eds. Rebecca L. Walker and Philip J. Ivanhoe (Oxford: Oxford University Press, 2007), 297–312, especially 303–305.
69. See for a moving testimony Andrew Bridge, *Hope's Boy* (New York: Hyperion, 2008), a memoir of his childhood in the foster care system. See in particular 295: "Love may not be enough to wake a child in the morning, dress him, and get him to school, then to feed him at night, bathe him, and put him to bed. Still, can any of us imagine a childhood without it?"
70. Compare Keller, *The Limits of Loyalty*, 125–126. See also Mills, "Duties to Aging Parents," 158–159.
71. See further Kupfer, "Can Parents and Children Be Friends?" Kupfer answers his question no, but claims that "the structural features which prevent complete friendship are also responsible for the . . . goods unique to parents and their adult children" (15).
72. See for an interesting though sometimes doleful discussion Ruth Padawer, "Losing Fatherhood," *New York Times Magazine*, November 22, 2009, 38ff.
73. Lauritzen, *Pursuing Parenthood*, 78, 79.
74. Tim Bayne, "Gamete Donation and Parental Responsibility," *Journal of Applied Philosophy* 20 (2003): 77–87, at 82.
75. Ibid., 83. Consistent with the claim that what procreators owe a child is to see to it that he or she is cared for, not necessarily to care for the child themselves, David Archard claims that, properly speaking, a procreator does not *alienate* but instead *discharges* his or her parental obligations in finding another individual or institution willing and able to care for the child. See Archard, "The Obligations and Responsibilities of Parenthood," in *Procreation and Parenthood*, 103–127, at 121.

76. Compare Nelson, "Parental Obligations and the Ethics of Surrogacy: A Causal Perspective," *Public Affairs Quarterly* 5 (1991): 49–61, at 60.

77. Compare Archard, "The Obligations and Responsibilities of Parenthood," 121, where he dismisses this "epistemic concern" as baseless. As Lauritzen notes, however, studies have found that birth mothers often worry nonetheless. See *Pursuing Parenthood*, 128–129.

78. Archard, "The Obligations of Parenthood," 121.

79. I thank a referee for this line of questioning.

80. See in this regard Stephanie Coontz, *The Social Origins of Private Life: A History of American Families 1600–1900* (London: Verso, 1988), 7–18; and "The Evolution of American Families," in *Families As They Really Are*, ed. Barbara J. Risman (New York: W.W. Norton, 2010), 30–47, especially 30–33.

81. Lauritzen, *Pursuing Parenthood*, 78.

82. The language of "abandonment" is Archard's; see "The Obligations and Responsibilities of Parenthood," 124.

83. Readers might recall the end of the book of Job, where the title character receives from God seven sons and three daughters to make up for the seven sons and three daughters lost, toward the beginning of the book, at the hands of Satan with God's complaisance.

NOTES TO CHAPTER 2

1. An exception is Archard, who distinguishes "the parental obligation" to ensure "*that* someone acts as a parent to the child" from "parental responsibilities" of "*acting as a parent*," which is to say rearing the child. See "The Obligations and Responsibilities of Parenthood," 104–105.

2. Judith Jarvis Thomson, "A Defense of Abortion," *Philosophy and Public Affairs* 1 (1971): 47–66, at 65. Compare Norman Daniels, "Duty to Treat or Right to Refuse?," *Hastings Center Report* 21/2 (1991): 36–46, at 44: "We have obligations to take certain risks only if we have consented to adopt those obligations and face those risks"—a claim sometimes taken to imply a thoroughgoing voluntarism about obligations. Contrast, however, Daniels's comments on the grounds of filial obligations in his *Am I My Parents' Keeper? An Essay on Justice between the Young and the Old* (Oxford: Oxford University Press, 1988), 29.

3. For such an argument, see Mills, "Duties to Aging Parents," 147–166. Mills agrees with Jane English that a grown child does not have a duty to "repay" his or her parents for debts incurred, but disagrees that the parent-child relationship is properly understood as a form of friendship. Whereas friends have duties to one another only so long as they remain friends—that is, only *within* the relationship—there is a case to be made that a grown child has a prima facie obligation to her parents to stay within, or at least seek to stay within, the relationship. Contrast Jane English, "What Do Grown Children Owe Their Parents?," in *Having Children: Philosophical and Legal Reflections on Parenthood*, eds. Onora O'Neill and William Ruddick (New York: Oxford University Press, 1979), 351–356.

4. Brake, "Willing Parents: A Voluntarist Account of Parental Role Obligations," in *Procreation and Parenthood*, 151–177, at 174.

5. Ibid.

6. Thomson, "A Defense of Abortion," 65.

7. Brake, "Fatherhood and Child Support," 59.

8. Archard, "The Obligations and Responsibilities of Parenthood," 105.
9. Ibid., 104.
10. Brake, "Willing Parents," 158.
11. Giuliana Fuscaldo, "Genetic Ties: Are They Morally Binding?," *Bioethics* 20 (2006): 64–76, at 67.
12. Fuscaldo, "Genetic Ties," 67.
13. Jeffrey Blustein, "Procreation and Parental Responsibility," *Journal of Social Philosophy* 28 (1997): 79–86, at 83.
14. Blustein, "Procreation and Parental Responsibility," 85. The claim that a child has a right to reasonable assurance of a decent life is derived from Joel Feinberg. See his "Wrongful Life and the Counterfactual Element in Harming," in *Freedom and Fulfillment: Philosophical Essays* (Princeton, NJ: Princeton University Press, 1992), 3–36, at 24–25.
15. Compare Nelson, "Parental Obligations and the Ethics of Surrogacy," 54–57. Contrast George Harris, "Fathers and Fetuses," *Ethics* 96 (1986): 594–603, at 597.
16. Brake, "Willing Parents," 156.
17. Diane Jeske, "Families, Friends, and Special Obligations," *Canadian Journal of Philosophy* 28 (1998): 527–556, at 529.
18. Michael O. Hardimon, "Role Obligations," *The Journal of Philosophy* 91 (1994): 333–363, at 357. Hardimon's examples of roles the acceptance of which is tacit include professor and doctor. Compare Brake, "Willing Parents," 170–171.
19. Hardimon, "Role Obligations," 347.
20. Ibid., 347–348. See for discussion A. John Simmons, "External Justifications and Institutional Roles," *Journal of Philosophy* 93 (1996): 28–36. Simmons focuses on the question of the normative independence of role obligations.
21. Brake, "Willing Parents," 171.
22. See Blustein, "Procreation and Parental Responsibility," 83–85; and Nelson, "Parental Obligations and the Ethics of Surrogacy," 54–57.
23. Brake, "Willing Parents," 157.
24. Ibid., 158.
25. Ibid., 160.
26. Ibid.
27. Ibid., 158.
28. Ibid., 155.
29. See again Blustein's "Procreation and Parental Responsibility," 85, as well as, more recently, his "Doing the Best for One's Child: Satisficing Versus Optimizing Parentalism," *Theoretical Medicine and Bioethics* 33 (2012): 199–205, at 201, where following Onora O'Neill he poses as "the parental sufficiency standard . . . an upbringing that brings up the child 'to at least the level which will minimally fit the child for independent adult life in its society.'" See O'Neill's "Begetting, Rearing, and Bearing," in *Having Children*, eds. O'Neill and Ruddick, 25–38, at 26.
30. Brake, "Willing Parents," 160.
31. Ibid., 160–161.
32. Ibid., 165–166.
33. Kant, *Metaphysik der Sitten*, ed. Karl Vorländer, 4th ed. (Hamburg: Felix Meiner, 1966), 6:281, p. 96; *The Metaphysics of Morals*, trans. Mary Gregor (Cambridge: Cambridge University Press, 1998), 64.
34. John Locke, *The Second Treatise of Government*, in *Two Treatises of Government*, ed. Peter Laslett (Cambridge: Cambridge University Press, 1988), §89, p. 207.

35. See here Archard, *Children: Rights and Childhood* (London: Routledge, 1993), 1–12, which is the book's first chapter, entitled "John Locke's Children."
36. Joseph Millum, "How Do We Acquire Parental Obligations?" *Social Theory and Practice* 34 (2008): 71–93, at 77.
37. Ibid.
38. Milton, *Paradise Lost*, bk. 10, lines 743–745, p. 236.
39. Ibid., lines 758–759, 762.
40. See Shelley, *Frankenstein*, 65, 98.
41. Ibid., 80, 81, 86.
42. Ibid., 80.
43. Ibid., 114.
44. Job 3:3–5 (NRSV).
45. See also Benatar's "Why It Is Better Never to Have Come into Existence," though, as noted already, I have serious reservations about the argument.
46. By the way, I have no interest here in denying the goodness of life itself or that some of the goods considered constitutive of it—Thomas Nagel lists perception, desire, activity, and thought—count as goods even though they are "conditions of misery as well as happiness," to quote from Nagel's famous paper on the badness of death. My question might then be restated: whether the goodness of life is good enough to justify giving it, whatever its conditions. As Nagel also notes, "a sufficient quantity of particular evils can perhaps outweigh" even the constitutive goods of life. See "Death," *Noûs* 4 (1970): 73–80, at 74.
47. Seana Valentine Shiffrin, "Wrongful Life, Procreative Responsibility, and the Significance of Harm," *Legal Theory* 5 (1999): 117–148, at 136.
48. See ibid., 137.
49. Ibid.
50. J. David Velleman, "Persons in Prospect," *Philosophy and Public Affairs* 36 (2008): 221–288, at 250. Velleman's account closely follows Shiffrin's, though he claims that parents cannot confer harms by bringing children into existence, and so what is equivocal about procreation is not that it harms the child, but more precisely "that it throws the child into a predicament, confronts it with a challenge in which the stakes are high, both for good and for ill" (251). I read Shiffrin as claiming, however, not that bringing a child into existence itself harms him or her, but that it exposes him or her to harms. On this reading, there seems very little if any difference between Shiffrin's and Velleman's accounts.
51. Shiffrin, "Wrongful Life, Procreative Responsibility, and the Significance of Harm," 133.
52. To draw this conclusion, Shiffrin invokes "the foundational liberal, antipaternalist principle that forbids the imposition of significant burdens and risks upon a person without the person's consent" and ascribes responsibility to agents who act contrary to this principle. See ibid., 139. To be clear, her position is not, as she emphasizes, "that procreation is all-things-considered wrong. . . . All I mean to advance," she writes, "is the claim that because procreation imposes a nonconsensual imposition of significant burdens, it is morally problematic and its imposer may justifiably he held responsible for its harmful results. . . . Thus, one might hold that the unconsented-to burdens of life do not make it wrong to procreate per se, but rather wrong to procreate without undertaking a commitment to share or alleviate any burdens the future child endures." See 139.
53. Compare Glover, *Choosing Children*, 52, which I have paraphrased.
54. Kant, *Metaphysik der Sitten*, 6:222, pp. 24–25; *The Metaphysics of Morals*, 15.

55. Shiffrin, "Wrongful Life, Procreative Responsibility, and the Significance of Harm," 140 (emphasis added).
56. It should be acknowledged that there could well be other grounds to justify saying no, if Frankenstein had conflicting duties of a sufficient seriousness. We would need to know the story here before being able to judge Frankenstein's obligations to the creature.
57. Shanley, "Fathers' Rights, Mothers' Wrongs?," 92.
58. By the way, I recognize that Frankenstein was not the creature's biological procreator, at least in the sense that the creature was not genetically derived from him. Arguably, however, Frankenstein—having, God-like, breathed life into the creature—had a yet more intimate bond with him than biological procreators do with offspring, mothers possibly excepted. Compare on this last point Genesis 4:1–2, where, as Robert Alter remarks, Eve presents herself as a "partner of God in man-making." See Alter's translation of *The Five Books of Moses* (New York: W. W. Norton, 2004), 29 (quoted with his permission).
59. See Millum, "How Do We Acquire Parental Obligations?," 77.
60. Compare Mills, "Duties to Aging Parents," 158–159, who claims moreover that grown children owe their parents "the very same thing," which is to say first and foremost "the relationship itself."
61. I take this phrase from Shakespeare's *King Lear*, 2.4.177.
62. Eugenio Montale, "Corno Inglese," from *Cuttlefish Bones*, in *Collected Poems 1920–1954*, trans. Jonathan Galassi, bilingual ed. (New York: Farrar, Straus and Giroux, 1998), 12, 13. The Italian is "*scordato strumento*" (12), translated by Galassi as "discordant instrument" (13).
63. In the *Groundwork*, which begins by insisting that the mark of a morally worthy action is that it is done purely "from duty," Kant claims that "love as an inclination cannot be commanded, but beneficence from duty itself, even though no inclination impels us to it and indeed natural and unconquerable aversion opposes it," can be commanded. For beneficence, he goes on, "is *practical* and not *pathological* love, which lies in the will and not in the propensity of feeling, in principles of action and not in melting sympathy." Similarly, in the *Critique of Practical Reason*, Kant claims that "love for God as inclination ([what he means by] pathological love) is not possible, for he is not an object of the senses," and that love of human beings "cannot be commanded, for it is not within the power of any human being to love someone simply on command." Once again, only "practical love" is possible, which Kant explicates here as striving to do our duties *gladly* (or *gerne*). See *Grundlegung zur Metaphysik der Sitten*, 4:99, p. 17; *Groundwork of the Metaphysics of Morals*, 13; and *Kritik der praktischen Vernunft*, ed. Horst D. Brandt and Heiner F. Klemme (Hamburg: Felix Meiner, 2003), 5:83, p. 112; *Critique of Practical Reason*, trans. Mary Gregor (Cambridge: Cambridge University Press, 1997), 71.
64. Compare Wilkinson, *Choosing Tomorrow's Children*, 23.
65. On this point, see Lawrence A. Blum, *Friendship, Altruism, and Morality* (London: Routledge, 1980), 13.
66. Alasdair MacIntyre, *Dependent Rational Animals: Why Human Beings Need the Virtues* (Chicago: Open Court, 1999), 122.
67. David Hume, *A Treatise of Human Nature*, ed. P.H. Nidditch, 2nd ed. (Oxford: Oxford University Press, 1978), bk. 3, pt. 2, §1, p. 479.
68. Liao, "The Idea of a Duty to Love," *The Journal of Value Inquiry* 40 (2006): 1–22, at 3. See also Keller, *The Limits of Loyalty*, 142–143.
69. Liao, "The Idea of a Duty to Love," 4.
70. Ibid., 4–5.

71. Ibid., 5.

72. Keller, *The Limits of Loyalty*, 143.

73. See, for example, the testimonial of Douglas Brown, "Good Practice for a Tough Fatherhood," *New York Times*, June 21, 2009, www.nytimes .com/2009/06/21/fashion/21love.html. Brown reflects on his struggles to learn to love his child Theo, who is autistic. We might also think of women who have suffered from postpartum depression or psychosis.

74. Hume, *Treatise*, bk. 3, pt. 2, §1, p. 478. Hume goes on from this point to claim that "it may be establish'd as an undoubted maxim, *that no action can be virtuous, or morally good, unless there be in human nature some motive to produce it, distinct from the sense of its morality*" (479)—a claim diametrically opposed to Kant's position in the first part of the *Groundwork*.

75. O'Neill, "The 'Good Enough' Parent in the Age of the New Reproductive Technologies," 37.

76. Compare Bettelheim, *A Good Enough Parent*, 75: "For a parent's love to be fully and positively effective it ought to be enlightened by thoughtfulness."

77. Kant, *Metaphysik der Sitten*, 6:399, p. 241; *The Metaphysics of Morals*, 159.

78. Robert Spaemann, *Persons: The Difference between 'Someone' and 'Something,'* trans. Oliver O'Donovan (Oxford: Oxford University Press, 2006), 215.

79. Kant, *Grundlegung*, 4:394, p. 11; *Groundwork*, 8.

80. Bernard Williams, "Moral Luck," in *Moral Luck: Philosophical Papers 1973–1980* (Cambridge: Cambridge University Press, 1981), 20–39, at 20–21. Elsewhere, Williams attacks the "transcendental psychology" that Kant develops in support of the view that "the source of moral thought and action must be located outside the empirically conditioned self." See "Morality and the Emotions," in *Problems of the Self: Philosophical Papers 1956–1972* (Cambridge: Cambridge University Press, 1973), 207–229, at 228.

81. Shakespeare, *King Lear*, 3.6.76–77.

82. Compare Spaemann, *Persons*, 20–21.

83. Blum, *Friendship, Altruism, and Morality*, 189.

84. At the same time, it should be acknowledged that becoming a parent, like other leaps in life, opens us to discoveries about ourselves, so judgments about who is fit to become a parent—even judgments about ourselves in this regard—should be made with great circumspection. See, for example, Harriet Brown, "A Family Label, Ungarbled," *New York Times*, February 28, 2010, www.nytimes.com/2010/02/28/fashion/28love.html. Brown begins her essay, "When I was pregnant for the first time, my biggest fear was not whether I would love the baby but whether I could."

85. See Scanlon, *What We Owe to Each Other* (Cambridge, MA: Harvard University Press, 1998), 173: Lacking affect "is not the whole of the problem. Affect is not a separable psychological element that might be added to the bare moral obligations . . . in order to produce an admirable parent. The lack of affect is a sign that the person . . . fails to see the good of being a parent—fails to see having children and caring for them as a way in which it is desirable to live."

86. I thank a referee for this observation.

87. Kant, *Grundlegung*, 4:389, p. 5; *Groundwork*, 2–3.

88. This claim might be supported by turning not only to Hume, but Aquinas. See in this regard Robert Miner, *Thomas Aquinas on the Passions: A Study of* Summa Theologiae *Ia2ae 22–48* (Cambridge: Cambridge University Press, 2009), 91–92 (especially n. 4) and 100–108.

89. A student of mine once commented in class discussion that she did not like her grandmother much at all, but still loved her. See also Richard A. Friedman, "Accepting That Good Parents May Plant Bad Seeds," *New York Times*, July 12, 2010, sec. D, recalling a former patient "who told me that she had given up trying to have a relationship with her 24-year-old daughter, whose relentless criticism she could no longer bear. 'I still love and miss her,' she said sadly. 'But I really don't like her.'"
90. Millum, "How Do We Acquire Parental Responsibilities?," 71.
91. Ibid., 75.
92. Ibid., 76.
93. Ibid., 88.
94. Ibid., 84, n. 35.
95. One last example: Millum writes that "gamete donors do not acquire parental responsibilities because their acts, though they may eventually lead to children, are not considered to constitute taking on responsibilities. (If gamete donors reasonably believe that they are not going to be held parentally responsible, then they have not taken on parental responsibilities by donating.)" See ibid., 79. "Considered" by whom and on what basis? "Reasonably" by what lights?

NOTES TO CHAPTER 3

1. Brake, "Fatherhood and Child Support," 63.
2. See David L. Chambers, "The Coming Curtailment of Compulsory Child Support," *Michigan Law Review* 80 (1982): 1614–1634, at 1619–1620.
3. On this point, see Lisa Sowle Cahill, "Abortion and Argument by Analogy," *Horizons* 9 (1982): 271–287, at 284.
4. Benatar, *Better Never to Have Been*, 33.
5. Cahill, "Abortion and Argument by Analogy," 284.
6. See, for example, Warren Quinn, "Abortion: Identity and Loss," *Philosophy and Public Affairs* 13 (1984): 24–54. It should also be noted, however, that Benatar rejects the "presumption in favour of continuing a pregnancy" and articulates instead what he calls "the 'pro-death' view," the conclusion of which is that "we should adopt a presumption, at least in the earlier stages of pregnancy, against carrying a fetus to term." His argument builds on two premises: (1) coming into existence is a harm (that is, *not* good and even bad), and (2) fetuses lack moral standing in at least the early stages of pregnancy. See *Better Never to Have Been*, 133 and 161. As noted in chapter 1, following no few others, I reject Benatar's thesis that nonexistence is better than existence. I do not then engage the pro-death view of abortion here—doing so would take us further into the literature on abortion than the project of this book has reason to go—but this view does deserve attention and a reply. Arguably, it may be consistent with and perhaps even the logical extension of an increasingly nonchalant attitude toward abortion—matters for a future paper to consider.
7. Brake, "Fatherhood and Child Support," 56.
8. Compare Millum, likewise drawing from Thomson's argument as precedent: "merely being the voluntary cause of the existence of a being with morally important needs is insufficient to give an agent a duty to meet those needs. Consequently, insofar as the duties of parents are duties to meet their children's morally important needs, they cannot derive simply from voluntarily causing their children to exist." See Millum's review of Michael W. Austin's *Conceptions of Parenthood: Ethics and the Family*

(Aldershot: Ashgate, 2007) for *Notre Dame Philosophical Reviews*, published April 26, 2008, http://ndpr.nd.edu/review.cfm?id=12946.

9. The director is Mel Feit, quoted by Nancy Gibbs in "A Man's Right to Choose?," *Time*, published online March 15, 2006, www.time.com/time/nation/article/0,8599,1173414,00.html. See for the Center's advocacy and arguments www.nationalcenterformen.org/. See also the case *Dubay v. Wells*, argued in the 6th Circuit U.S. Court of Appeals in 2007, dubbed "*Roe v. Wade* for Men," with which the Center was involved.

10. Keith J. Pavlischek, "Abortion Logic and Paternal Responsibilities: One More Look at Judith Thomson's 'A Defense of Abortion,'" *Public Affairs Quarterly* 7 (1993): 341–361, at 349.

11. Ibid., 343.

12. Ibid., 342.

13. For an excellent discussion, see Shelley Burtt, "Reproductive Responsibilities: Rethinking the Fetal Rights Debate," *Policy Sciences* 27 (1994): 179–196.

14. Brake, "Fatherhood and Child Support," 68. To be fair, Brake may mean that, if adoption is permissible, the causal account of parental obligations is "clearly false" because adoption allows parents to alienate or disclaim parental rights and obligations in the expectation or hope that they will be transferred to others who may or may not be biologically related to the children in question. See ibid., 56. Brake ignores here, however, the question of whether parental obligations can be legitimately alienated or transferred under all circumstances, or only when there are good reasons. See chapters 1 and 2.

15. For this claim, see Millum, "How Do We Acquire Parental Responsibilities?," 74, n. 9.

16. As Brake remarks, "It seems difficult to impute tacit consent [to parental obligations] to someone who intended to avoid pregnancy, simply because he or she knew of the possibility. . . . [S]urely consent, to be a meaningful moral concept, must be something more than foresight." And Nelson agrees: "True, [the unwilling father] engaged in sexual intercourse knowing there was some slim chance that . . . contraceptives would fail, but to construe that as choosing to accept responsibility for any child that does ensue is to strain the notion of choice to the breaking point. All of us engage in activities which have foreseeable risks; that does not imply that we agree to accept responsibility for those risks should they materialize." See Brake, "Fatherhood and Child Support," 60; and Nelson, "Parental Obligations and the Ethics of Surrogacy," 55.

17. Nelson, "Parental Obligations and the Ethics of Surrogacy," 60.

18. Brake, "Fatherhood and Child Support," 56.

19. Thomson, "A Defense of Abortion," 48.

20. A referee has suggested the following, admittedly rough analogy: suppose one has a backyard pool, and there is a child in the neighborhood who is a poor swimmer. One tells his parents that he is invited to swim in the pool this afternoon, at a time when they can't be present. With this invitation, one incurs a responsibility to keep a close eye on the child—but only should his parents permit him to come over to swim. Otherwise one certainly would not have any such responsibility, which is then contingent on the parents' decision, which one cannot force either way. But if they did accept the invitation—that is, if they followed through—then one's responsibility would follow as well.

21. Brake, "Fatherhood and Child Support," 58.

22. Thomson, "A Defense of Abortion," 59.

23. Ibid.

24. It might be countered, as Brake anticipates, that the "differential burdens" of pregnancy, on the one hand, and child support, on the other, justify recognizing that women have a right to abortion, while denying that men have a corresponding right to free themselves from parental obligations. In its simplest form, the argument claims that childbearing and paying child support just do not compare—childbearing poses risks and imposes burdens that paying child support just does not—and so it is no injustice for women, but not men, to have the choice whether to support a child (granting at least for the sake of argument that a fetus has the same moral standing). Compare Laura Purdy, "Abortion and the Husband's Rights: A Reply to Wesley Teo," *Ethics* 86 (1976): 247–251, at 250. Brake replies that "the different burdens argument ignores the realities of many men's lives" and that, "[i]n some cases, compelling child support may unacceptably diminish men's autonomy." See Brake, "Fatherhood and Child Support," 65 and 66. I agree with Brake that the current child support system in the United States has much room for improvement, but to agree that the public has significant responsibility for children's welfare is not also to agree that so-called unwilling fathers do not themselves bear some measure of such responsibility and so should not be required to make even a small payment. Compare Chambers, "Fathers, the Welfare System, and the Virtues and Perils of Child-Support Enforcement," *Virginia Law Review* 81 (1995): 2575–2605, at 2594–2596.

25. Brake, "Fatherhood and Child Support," 56.

26. Ibid., 58.

27. Thomson, "A Defense of Abortion," 65.

28. Thomson asserts that resort to abortion "may be positively indecent" in some cases—for example, if a woman "is in her seventh month, and wants the abortion just to avoid the nuisance of postponing a trip abroad"—but notoriously gives no criteria to determine what would count as "decent" and what "indecent," and what's more provides no framework for considering this indecency as any worse than *distasteful*. If morality reduces to respecting liberty rights—Thomson's libertarian creed—what could be *morally* wrong about indecency? See ibid., 65–66. See further in this regard O'Neill, *Towards Justice and Virtue: A Constructive Account of Practical Reasoning* (Cambridge: Cambridge University Press, 1996), 142–146; and "The Great Maxims and Justice and Charity," in her *Constructions of Reason: Explorations of Kant's Practical Philosophy* (Cambridge: Cambridge University Press, 1989), 219–233.

29. Brake, "Willing Parents," 14. It is, however, worth noting that, should the child's parents not themselves care for his or her needs and instead abandon the child, they would wrong not only the child but those upon the prima facie duty of rescue would then fall in the case that these persons were not responsible for the child's coming into being.

30. N. Ann Davis, "Fiddling Second: Reflections on 'A Defense of Abortion,'" in *Fact and Value: Essays on Ethics and Metaphysics for Judith Jarvis Thomson*, eds. Alex Byrne, Robert Stalnaker, and Ralph Wedgwood (Cambridge, MA: The MIT Press, 2001), 81–96, at 93.

31. Thomson, "A Defense of Abortion," 49.

32. See Christopher Kaczor, *The Ethics of Abortion: Women's Rights, Human Life, and the Question of Justice* (Routledge: New York, 2011), 152–153, for accounts of suction curettage, dilation and evacuation, dilation and extraction, and induction.

33. See Francis J. Beckwith, "Personal Bodily Rights, Abortion, and Unplugging the Violinist," *International Philosophical Quarterly* 32 (1992): 105–118, at 116, citing discussions by Baruch Brody, Stephen D. Schwarz, and R.K. Tacelli.
34. See, for example, Mary Anne Warren, "On the Moral and Legal Status of Abortion," *The Monist* 57 (1973): 43–61, at 49–50.
35. Jeff McMahan, *The Ethics of Killing: Problems at the Margins of Life* (Oxford: Oxford University Press, 2002), 383, which I have paraphrased.
36. James Rachels, "Active and Passive Euthanasia," *New England Journal of Medicine* 292 (1975): 78–80.
37. Ludwig Wittgenstein, *Philosophical Investigations*, trans. G.E.M. Anscombe, 2nd, bilingual ed. (Oxford: Basil Blackwell, 1958), §66, p. 32. Compare Tom L. Beauchamp and James F. Childress, *Principles of Biomedical Ethics*, 6th ed. (Oxford: Oxford University Press, 2009), 172–174.
38. McMahan, *The Ethics of Killing*, 384.
39. Ibid., 382.
40. Ibid., 384.
41. Ibid., 386. Contrast Philippa Foot, "The Problem of Abortion and the Doctrine of the Double Effect," in *Virtues and Vices and Other Essays in Moral Philosophy* (Berkeley: University of California Press, 1978), 19–32, at 26, where she claims that "the root idea" of allowing to die is "the removal of some obstacle which is, as it were, holding back a train of events."
42. McMahan, *The Ethics of Killing*, 386.
43. Ibid., 388.
44. Ibid., 383.
45. Foot, "The Problem of Abortion and the Doctrine of the Double Effect," 26. I am aware, by the way, that it might be objected that whether parents' failing to feed their child is categorized as killing or letting die is of no matter, since, for any given description of the distinction between killing and letting die, the distinction makes no necessary difference in judgments about moral culpability, such that both cases of killing and cases of letting die may be judged cases of murder. I agree, but I also think that categorizing cases of murder as killing is more consistent not only with ordinary language, but with the law of homicide. To be clear, I am not thereby committing myself to the thesis that every case of killing (or homicide) is a case of murder. Instead, I hold that every case of murder can rightly and sensibly be called a case of killing (homicide), in particular, culpable killing.
46. Richard A. McCormick, "Vive la Différence! Killing and Allowing to Die," *America*, December 6, 1997, 6–12, at 9.
47. See McMahan, *The Ethics of Killing*, 386.
48. See Foot, "Killing and Letting Die," in *Moral Dilemmas and Other Topics in Moral Philosophy* (Oxford: Oxford University Press, 2002), 78–87, at 87, where she writes that "what matters" when we exculpate someone for the death of another on the grounds that this other has been allowed to die is not whether or not "the use of 'kill'" would be appropriate, but "that the fatal sequence resulting in death is not initiated but is rather allowed to take its course." Foot does not claim, however, that initiating a fatal sequence of events *external* to an individual's natural state is necessary for us to speak of killing.
49. This is not, by the way, a definition of killing, but a characterization of one form of it.

50. Foot, "The Problem of Abortion and the Doctrine of the Double Effect," 26–27 and 29. See also "Killing and Letting Die," 79.

51. McMahan acknowledges that "[t]here is, of course, a temptation to say that parents who fail to feed their baby thereby kill it." He dismisses this "temptation," however, with the claim that it "can readily be explained by reference to our desire to condemn the parents in the strongest possible terms," which we are led to do, according to him, because "the wrongfulness of allowing the child to die is magnified by the way in which one is related to the child," namely, here as his or her parent. See *The Ethics of Killing*, 386 and 236–237. This highly speculative claim, however, makes no sense of my "temptation" to say that the fish's caretaker and the boater did not merely let the individual in question die, but in a sense killed it and him or her—the sense of killing that does not involve the initiation of a sequence of threatening events, but does involve withholding or withdrawing life support, such that this withholding or withdrawal ultimately causes the death.

52. This case too, however, could be categorized as killing if it were judged that the person to whom the violinist had been connected had a strict duty to him not to let him die. But this judgment seems baseless as Thomson tells the story.

53. For such a discussion, see Rosalind Hursthouse, "Virtue Theory and Abortion," *Philosophy and Public Affairs* 20 (1991): 223–246, at 237–238, which I paraphrase. I would place more importance than Hursthouse does, however, on considerations of the status of the fetus, which she dismisses as more or less "irrelevant" (see 235–236). Contrast in this regard Quinn, "Abortion: Identity and Loss."

54. For a quite interesting history of this development, see Hansen, "The American Invention of Child Support."

55. A third possible focus, it should be noted, is on fetuses that women have decided to carry to term. See, again, Burtt, "Reproductive Responsibilities: Rethinking the Fetal Rights Debate."

56. Brake, "Fatherhood and Child Support," 60, quoting David Boonin, *A Defense of Abortion* (Cambridge: Cambridge University Press, 2002), 171. Compare Millum, "How Do We Acquire Parental Responsibilities?," 77.

57. Harry S. Silverstein, "On a Woman's 'Responsibility' for the Fetus," *Social Theory and Practice* 13 (1987): 103–119, at 110.

58. See for development ibid., 106–109; and Boonin, "A Defense of 'A Defense of Abortion': On the Responsibility Objection to Thomson's Argument," *Ethics* 107 (1997): 286–313, at 301–306.

59. McMahan, *The Ethics of Killing*, 366–367. As McMahan writes further, it seems that Silverstein's argument "conflates the impossibility of preventing an individual from being in a certain state with the impossibility of preventing the individual from being in that state, *given that he exists*" (367).

60. Pavlischek, "Abortion Logic and Paternal Responsibilities," 343.

61. Padawer, "Losing Fatherhood," 41.

62. See ibid. Padawer discusses cases in Pennsylvania, Florida, and Georgia.

63. Ibid., 62, characterizing the thinking of Pennsylvania judge David Wecht.

NOTES TO CHAPTER 4

1. See, for example, Justice William Brennan's Opinion of the Court in *Eisenstadt v. Baird*: "If the right to privacy means anything, it is the right of the individual, married or single, to be free from unwanted government intrusion into matters so fundamentally affecting a person as the decision whether to bear or beget a child" (405 U.S. 438, 453 [1972]). As former

solicitor general Charles Fried has observed, drawing attention to both the use of the term 'individual' and the reference to childbearing, "Thus was the seed planted from which *Roe* grew," or more precisely what Justice Harry Blackmun called in that decision "a right of personal privacy, or a guarantee of certain areas or zones of privacy," which he located primarily in the Fourteenth Amendment's Due Process Clause and judged to be "broad enough to encompass a woman's decision whether or not to terminate her pregnancy" (410 U.S. 113, 152, 153 [1973]). See Charles Fried, *Order and Law: Arguing the Reagan Revolution—A Firsthand Account* (New York: Simon & Schuster, 1991), 77. For an extensive discussion of the relevant jurisprudence, see I. Glenn Cohen, "The Constitution and the Rights Not to Procreate," *Stanford Law Review* 60 (2008): 1135–1196, especially 1148–1167, analyzing the U.S. Supreme Court's contraception and abortion cases.

2. It might be objected that traditional surrogacy has a long and even august history, reaching all the way back to the book of Genesis and the story of Abraham's impregnation of Sarah's slave Hagar, leading to the birth of Ishmael. There are significant differences, however, between surrogacy as represented in Genesis and the contemporary practice. Whereas the contemporary practice is sometimes celebrated as having "the potential to empower women," as Laura Purdy claims, by contrast, in Genesis it was because Hagar was Sarah's slave and, as such, "at her disposal," as Oliver O'Donovan puts it, that Hagar was a fitting replacement for Sarah. It should also be noted that the Genesis story does not have the happiest of endings. After conceiving Ishmael, Hagar looks down upon Sarah—"her mistress seemed slight in her eyes" (Genesis 16:5)—thereby refusing her subordination and, again to quote O'Donovan, "asserting herself as mother in her own right." The upshot is that "the representational arrangement collapsed and the child Ishmael was disowned." See Purdy, "Surrogate Mothering: Exploitation or Empowerment?" *Bioethics* 3 (1989): 18–34, at 34; and Oliver O'Donovan, *Begotten or Made?* (Oxford: Oxford University Press, 1984), 34. The biblical translation is from Robert Alter's *The Five Books of Moses*, 78 (quoted with his permission).

3. See Robin Marantz Henig, *Pandora's Baby: How the First Test Tube Babies Sparked the Reproductive Revolution* (Boston: Houghton Mifflin, 2004).

4. It should be noted that the official teaching of the Roman Catholic Church rules out all techniques of assisted reproduction that "substitute for the conjugal act" or "dissociate procreation from the integrally personal context of the conjugal act"; see, for example, the 2008 instruction *Dignitatis personae*, §§12 and 16. See for discussion and a response to this teaching Lauritzen, *Pursuing Parenthood*, 3–14.

5. See Alex Kuczynski, "Her Body, My Baby," *New York Times Magazine*, November 30, 2008, 42ff., at 48 and 49, quoting the woman whom Kuczynski and her husband chose to carry an embryo produced by her egg and her husband's sperm. Kuczynski likens gestational surrogacy to "organ rental" (46) and is emphatic that the surrogate was a mere vessel for "our baby—coming out of her body" (78). The surrogate helps with this interpretation.

6. See Elizabeth S. Anderson, "Is Women's Labor a Commodity?" *Philosophy and Public Affairs* 19 (1990): 71–92, at 83.

7. Krimmel, "The Case against Surrogate Parenting," 35.

8. Anderson, "Is Women's Labor a Commodity?," 81–82.

9. Susan Moller Okin, *Women in Western Political Thought* (Princeton, NJ: Princeton University Press, 1979), 82, 82–83 for discussion and citations. See further Jane Maienschein, *Whose View of Life? Embryos, Cloning and Stem Cells* (Cambridge, MA: Harvard University Press, 2003), 13–16.
10. Richard Lewontin, *The Triple Helix: Gene, Organism, and Environment* (Cambridge, MA: Harvard University Press, 2000), 5.
11. Ibid., 6.
12. Compare Debrah Satz, *Why Some Things Should Not Be for Sale: The Moral Limits of Markets* (Oxford: Oxford University Press, 2010), 131, who comments that, when "[g]enes alone are taken to define natural and biological motherhood," the upshot is that "women's contribution to reproduction is recognized only insofar as it is identical to that of men" and "an old stereotype of women as merely the incubators of men's seeds" is reinforced.
13. See, for example, Scott F. Gilbert, "When 'Personhood' Begins in the Embryo: Avoiding a Syllabus of Errors," *Birth Defects Research* 84/Part C (2008): 164–173.
14. See Tim Bayne and Avery Kolers, "'Are You My Mommy?' On the Genetic Basis of Parenthood," *Journal of Applied Philosophy* 18 (2001): 273–285, at 279–280, who go on to criticize this argument.
15. Ibid., 280.
16. See Bayne and Kolers, "Toward a Pluralist Account of Parenthood," *Bioethics* 17 (2003): 221–242, at 229, who go on to criticize this argument as well.
17. Ibid., 230.
18. By the way, I put aside for now—and until chapter 5—the question of the grounds of parental rights; the focus of this chapter is again on the grounds of parental obligations.
19. H.L.A. Hart, *The Concept of Law* (Oxford: Oxford University Press, 1961), 119–120; see also the famous example on 125–126 of the concept 'vehicle' and the rule "no vehicle to be taken into the park."
20. Archard, "The Obligations and Responsibilities of Parenthood," 112–113.
21. Ibid., 113. Archard has in view Austin, *Conceptions of Parenthood*, 53.
22. See Joseph Millum's review of Austin's book for *Notre Dame Philosophical Reviews*, http://ndpr.nd.edu/review.cfm?id=12946.
23. See for discussion of the mixed motives of providers Thomas H. Murray, "New Reproductive Technologies and the Family," in *New Ways of Making Babies: The Case of Egg Donation*, ed. Cynthia B. Cohen (Bloomington: Indiana University Press, 1996), 51–69, at 62–63. Murray discusses both sperm and egg providers, whom he claims in some cases may rightly be called donors, in other cases more properly vendors.
24. Compare Suzanne Holland, "Contested Commodities at Both Ends of Life: Buying and Selling Gametes, Embryos, and Body Tissues," *Kennedy Institute of Ethics Journal* 11 (2001): 263–284, at 274.
25. See in this regard Aaron D. Levine, "Self-Regulation, Compensation, and the Ethical Recruitment of Oocyte Donors," *Hastings Center Report* 40/2 (2010): 25–36.
26. Benatar, "The Unbearable Lightness of Bringing into Being," *Journal of Applied Philosophy* 16 (1999): 173–180, at 176. Compare Weinberg, "The Moral Complexity of Sperm Donation," 172–173.
27. Brake, "Fatherhood and Child Support," 68. See also Millum, "How Do We Acquire Parental Responsibilities?," 72, n. 3.
28. Bayne, "Gamete Donation and Parental Responsibility," 79.
29. Ibid.

30. Fuscaldo, "Genetic Ties," 73.
31. Ibid., 74.
32. Nelson, "Parental Obligations and the Ethics of Surrogacy," 54. Nelson classifies gamete providers as surrogates; see 57.
33. Ibid., 54.
34. McMahan, *The Ethics of Killing*, 226.
35. I follow McMahan here, though he speculates that the "bare genetic relation" might somehow generate special responsibility. See ibid., 376. See further Niko Kolodny, "Which Relationships Justify Partiality? The Case of Parents and Children," *Philosophy and Public Affairs* 38 (2010): 37–75, at 61–75.
36. See Shiffrin, "Wrongful Life, Procreative Responsibility, and the Significance of Harm," 144.
37. Cynthia B. Cohen, "Parents Anonymous," in *New Ways of Making Babies*, 88–105, at 96.
38. Ibid.
39. See Donagan, *The Theory of Morality*, 160.
40. See for discussion ibid., 43–48. It might be asked, however, whether these two qualifications suffice. As a referee noted, "Some consequences of an action, although not abnormal and not mediated by the actions of others, do not reasonably seem to be part of the action itself. For example, bringing people into existence can reliably be expected to result in the death of those brought into existence. Yet, it doesn't seem to be the case that an act of procreation is also an act of killing." To reply to this example, certainly bringing into being is not killing, but it is subjecting one to death—which I then would be willing to count as part of the action. This consideration, among others, underlies Shiffrin's "equivocal view" of procreation discussed in chapter 2: namely, that being brought into being is a mixed benefit, compromised by significant and inevitable burdens. I believe that I would reply similarly to other counterexamples to the account of action in question.
41. For this example, see I. Glenn Cohen, "The Right Not to Be a Genetic Parent?" *Southern California Law Review* 81 (2008): 1115–1196, at 117, a "fact pattern" derived from the 2005 Illinois case of *Phillips v. Irons*.
42. See, again, Kolodny, "Which Relationships Justify Partiality?," 61–75. Contrast Christine Overall, *Why Have Children? The Ethical Debate* (Cambridge, MA: The MIT Press, 2012), 45–46, who holds that "the fact that a man does not anticipate a pregnancy as a result of oral sex is not a defense," since "we have a greater responsibility to be careful with our gametes than with our other bodily parts and fluids" (45). I generally agree with the claim in the last clause, but there is a logical gap, which Overall does not fill, between this claim and the conclusion that "the inseminator should be responsible, to the extent he is able, for contributing to [the resulting child's] support" (46). The child's need for care might well lead a compassionate man—but a court?—to this conclusion; the greater responsibility that we have for our gametes than we generally do for, say, our urine, saliva, or blood does not. Overall comes to the same conclusion in the further case of a man who needs to give a sperm sample to a laboratory and asks a female acquaintance to store it for him overnight in her refrigerator—only for her to use it for her own purposes. Change the terms of the case: let's say that one's blood poses a serious health risk to others. Then one would have a great responsibility to be careful with one's blood. One needs to give a blood sample to a laboratory and asks an acquaintance to store it overnight in her refrigerator—only

for her to use it to infect others. Would one be morally responsible for these infections? I think that the answer is surely no.

43. 2 Samuel 11:1, translated by Robert Alter in *The David Story* (New York: W. W. Norton, 1999), 250. I quote from Alter's translation (with his permission) in the following.

44. 2 Samuel 11:11, p. 252.

45. 2 Samuel 11:15, p. 253.

46. 2 Samuel 12:5–7, pp. 258–259.

47. Shiffrin, "Wrongful Life, Procreative Responsibility, and the Significance of Harm," 147, from which also come the following quotations in the paragraph. Shiffrin then agrees with the "rationale . . . voiced" in *Johnson v. Calvert*, 851 P.2d 776 (Ca. 1993), but does not follow the court in holding that the gestational surrogate is not a "natural mother," or more precisely that intention decides this question. See 147, n. 58.

48. At the same time, as the dissenting judge noted in *Johnson v. Calvert*, 851 P.2d 776, 799, "It requires little imagination to foresee cases in which the genetic mothers are, for example, unstable or substance abusers, or in which the genetic mothers' life circumstances change dramatically during the gestational mothers' pregnancy, while the gestational mothers, though of a less advantaged socioeconomic class, are stable, mature, capable and willing to provide a loving family environment in which the child will flourish."

49. For example, the intended father in *Stiver v. Parker*, 975 F.2d 261 (6th Cir. 1992), effectively abandoned the child, thought at first to be his genetically, when he was born with disabilities.

50. See on this point Annie Murphy Paul, *Origins: How the Nine Months before Birth Shape the Rest of Our Lives* (New York: Free Press, 2010), especially 5–7; and David H. Barad and Brian L. Cohen, "Oocyte Donation Program at Montefiore Medical Center, Albert Einstein," in *New Ways of Making Babies*, 15–28, at 26: "the gestational mother is not a passive vessel, but an active force in the creation of a new life."

51. See *In re Baby M*, 537 A.2d 1227 (N.J. 1988) and *A.G.R. v. D.R.H. & S.H.*, No. FD-09–1838–07 (N.J. Super. Ct. Chi. Div., Dec. 23, 2009).

52. By way of example, in *Donovan v. Idant Laboratories*, 625 F. Supp. 2d 256 (E.D. PA 2009), the court initially ruled that Idant, a sperm bank, was subject to strict products liability for having failed to detect genetic defects in a provider's sperm. The suit, however, was later thrown out on the grounds that it was essentially a claim for wrongful life, not a legally cognizable cause of action under New York law. In 1991, Idant came to an out-of-court settlement with Julia Skolnick, who had sued the sperm bank and Dr. Hugh Melnick of Advanced Fertility Services for having mistakenly inseminated her with the sperm of a black man rather than her white, deceased husband. See here Ronald Sullivan, "Sperm Mix-Up Lawsuit Is Settled," *New York Times*, August 1, 1991, sec. A.

53. Shelley, *Frankenstein*, 67; see also 151. The creature comes to life "on a dreary night of November" (see 34); Victor first feels the duties of a creator in August of the next year (67).

54. Bayne, "Gamete Donation and Parental Responsibility," 82.

55. Ibid., 83.

56. Lisa Sowle Cahill, "Moral Concerns about Institutionalized Gamete Donation," in *New Ways of Making Babies*, 70–87, at 77.

57. Compare Heidi Malm, "Paid Surrogacy: Arguments and Responses," *Public Affairs Quarterly* 3 (1989): 57–64, at 63.

58. Austin, *Conceptions of Parenthood*, 53.

59. See Ross, *The Right and the Good*, 19. Beauchamp and Childress, *Principles of Biomedical Ethics*, 15: "A *prima facie* obligation is one that must be fulfilled unless it conflicts, on a particular occasion, with an equal or stronger obligation. This type of obligation is always binding *unless* a competing moral obligation outweighs it in a particular circumstance."

60. See in this regard Lauritzen, *Pursuing Parenthood*, ix–xiii and xx.

61. For what it's worth, for my own take on double-effect reasoning, see "Double Effect, All Over Again: The Case of Sister Margaret McBride," *Theoretical Medicine and Bioethics* 32 (2011): 271–283.

62. McCormick, "Ambiguity in Moral Choice," in *Doing Evil to Achieve Good: Moral Choice in Conflict Situations*, eds. Richard A. McCormick, S.J., and Paul Ramsey (Chicago: Loyola University Press, 1978), 7–53, at 45.

63. Ibid.

64. See Lauritzen, *Pursuing Parenthood*, 128. Cahill replies in her "Moral Concerns about Institutionalized Gamete Donation," 81–83. See further, for a moving and thoughtful discussion, John Seabrook, "The Last Babylift: Adopting a Child in Haiti," *The New Yorker*, May 10, 2010, 44–53.

65. Daniel Callahan, "Bioethics and Fatherhood," *Utah Law Review* 3 (1992): 735–746, at 743, 745. He goes on: "there is something symbolically destructive about using anonymous sperm donors to help women have children apart from a permanent marital relationship with the father. For what action could more decisively declare the irrelevance of fatherhood than a specific effort to keep everyone ignorant?" (745).

66. Anderson, "Is Women's Labor a Commodity?," 90.

67. See, for example, Richard J. Arneson, "Commodification and Commercial Surrogacy," *Philosophy and Public Affairs* 21 (1992): 132–164, at 142: "Market trading in parental rights and duties will take place at the margin, not at the center, of childbearing practices."

68. Page, "Donation, Surrogacy and Adoption," 168.

69. It could be objected here that permitting donation to a *single* intended parent is wrong because, on the whole, children raised in single-parent households suffer significant deprivations compared to children raised in two-parent households (whatever the parents' genders). The objection seems to me important, and I leave the question open for empirical argumentation.

70. Elizabeth Marquardt, Norval D. Glenn, and Karen Clark, *My Daddy's Name Is Donor: A New Study of Young Adults Conceived through Sperm Donation* (New York: Institute for American Values, 2010), 5. It should be noted, however, that this study has provoked controversy on account both of its methodology and its political affiliation.

71. Ibid., 9.

72. Ibid., 11–12. Countries that have banned anonymous donation of sperm and eggs include the United Kingdom, Sweden, Norway, the Netherlands, and Switzerland (12).

73. Ibid., 13–14.

74. See, for example, the contributions of Diane B. Kunz, Arthur Caplan, Charles P. Kindregan, Jr., and Rebecca Dresser to the online discussion "The Baby Market," *New York Times*, December 29, 2009, http://room fordebate.blogs.nytimes.com/2009/12/29/the-baby-market/. As Caplan remarks in his contribution, "Ethics and Fees," "There are more laws in the United States governing the breeding of dogs, cats, fish, exotic animals, and wild game species than exist with respect to the use of surrogates and reproductive technologies to make people." In February 2008,

the American Bar Association published its "Model Act for Governing Assisted Reproductive Technology"; see www.abanet.org/family/commit tees/artmodelact.pdf. The adoption of this act by state legislatures would represent progress, but according to the argument that I have developed there would be reason to hope for further progress yet. For example, the model act permits provider anonymity "so long as non-identifying health information is provided" (article 2, section 204)—better, but not good enough.

75. For this worry, see Purdy, "At the Crossroads," 306.
76. See Callahan, "Bioethics and Fatherhood," 740–741. Compare O'Donovan, *Begotten or Made?*, 10–11, on "the exclusive importance of compassion among the virtues" in much contemporary thought.
77. Compare Austin, *Conceptions of Parenthood*, 53.
78. Shiffrin, "Wrongful Life, Procreative Responsibility, and the Significance of Harm," 145. It should be noted that Shiffrin holds, as I do not, that "biological parents remain susceptible for support payments." In the sentence that I have quoted in the body of my text, it is this support requirement that she suggests ought to be waived in order to facilitate adoptions.
79. See in this regard Ferdinand Schoeman, "Rights of Children, Rights of Parents, and the Moral Basis of the Family," *Ethics* 91 (1980): 6–19, at 14–19. Compare Francis Schrag's quite interesting "Justice and the Family," *Inquiry* 19 (1976): 193–208, at 203–207.
80. Compare Ken Daniels, "The Semen Providers," in *Donor Insemination: International Social Science Perspectives*, eds. Ken Daniels and Erica Haimes (Cambridge: Cambridge University Press, 1998), 76–104, at 96: "The semen provider gives a core part of himself through his semen; it could be said that he is in effect giving himself. In this respect he is very different from a blood donor or an organ donor. These people certainly provide a part of themselves, but that part is of a different order in that it enables another life to be maintained, rather than created."
81. Wittgenstein, *Philosophical Investigations*, pt. 1, §123, p. 49.
82. *In re Baby M*, 537 A.2d 1227, 1249 (N.J. 1988).
83. For a disturbing discussion, see Stephanie Saul, "Building a Baby, with Few Ground Rules," *New York Times*, December 13, 2009, sec. A, available online at www.nytimes.com/2009/12/13/us/13surrogacy.html.
84. See Charles P. Kindegran, Jr., "Licenses for Surrogacy Clinics," in "The Baby Market," http://roomfordebate.blogs.nytimes.com/2009/12/29/ the-baby-market/. See also the ABA model act, article 7, section 703, mandating, "[u]nless waived by the court," that "the relevant child-welfare agency" make "a home-study of the intended parents" and verify that the intended parents "meet the standards of suitability applicable to adoptive parents."
85. As the American College of Obstetricians and Gynecologists (ACOG) has observed, "In some states [in the U.S.], the practice of surrogate motherhood is not clearly covered under the law," such that it is unclear how surrogate contracts would fare. Further, "[t]here is a split among states that have statutes. Some states prohibit surrogate contracts [for example, Michigan] or make them void and unenforceable [for example, New Jersey], whereas others permit such agreements [for example, California and Texas]." See "Surrogate Motherhood," ACOG Committee Opinion No. 397, *Obstetrics & Gynecology* 111 (2008): 465–470, at 365. For an overview of state laws, see the "Guide to State Surrogacy Laws" compiled by the Center for American Progress and published December 17, 2007 online at www .americanprogress.org/issues/2007/12/surrogacy_laws.html. For a survey

of laws globally, see chapter 15 of the IFFS Surveillance 2010, eds. Howard Jones, Ian Cooke, Roger Kempers, Peter Brinsden, and Doug Saunders, published online by *Fertility and Sterility* at www.iffs-reproduction.org/documents/IFFS_Surveillance_2010.pdf.

86. Anderson, "Is Women's Labor a Commodity?," 92. For her definition of commodity, see 72.
87. Ibid., 81.
88. See ibid., 90, quoted above.
89. Ibid., 82.
90. Ibid., 89.
91. For an interesting discussion, see Paul, *Origins*, 150–151, on the mid-twentieth century research of Grete Lehner Bibring on the psychology of pregnancy; and 234–235, on contemporary research on so-called maternal programming: "the possibility that the physiological changes of pregnancy prime a woman's brain for parenting, that pregnancy grows not just a baby but a mother" (235).
92. See Anderson, "Is Women's Labor a Commodity?," 81–84. It should be noted that Satz has criticized Anderson's argument as turning on "the *essentialist thesis*" that "reproductive labor is by its nature something that should not be sold." I do not think, however, that Satz has Anderson right. According to Satz, what Anderson sees as wrong about surrogacy is that a woman's "selling her reproductive labor alienates [her] from her 'normal' and justified emotions." Satz counters that "not all women bond with their fetuses. Some women abort them." And she asks further, "Are we really sure that we know which emotions pregnancy 'normally' involves?" See *Why Some Things Should Not Be for Sale*, 117, 121, 122. But we need not understand Anderson as committed to a thesis about the "nature" of women's reproductive labor in all contexts, or as claiming that a woman will "normally" develop emotional ties to the child she is carrying irrespective of social practices surrounding pregnancy. Anderson's point is that, at least in most contemporary cultures, pregnancy is surrounded by social practices that encourage bonding. What is more, there is surely good reason to value these practices, though no doubt some can be criticized on feminist grounds (as no doubt others can be defended on feminist grounds.) Satz claims that "[t]he problem with commodifying women's reproductive labor is not that it degrades the special nature of reproductive labor . . ., but that it reinforces . . . a traditional gender-hierarchical division of labor. A consequence of my argument is that under very different background conditions, such contracts would be less objectionable" (*Why Some Things Should Not Be for Sale*, 131). Anderson could certainly agree with the claim of this last sentence: for her too, it is the "background conditions" of pregnancy that make commercial surrogacy so problematic. But she holds that there is reason to value (at least some of) these conditions.
93. *In re Baby M*, 537 A.2d 1227, 1248 (N.J. 1988).
94. Andrews, "Surrogate Motherhood," 74, 75. For discussion of "fertility tourism," see Jennifer Rimm, "Booming Baby Business: Regulating Commercial Surrogacy in India," *University of Pennsylvania Journal of International Law* 30 (2008–2009): 1429–1462, especially 1443–1446 and 1451–1452; and Judith Warner, "Outsourced Wombs," *New York Times*, online, January 3, 2008, at http://opinionator.blogs.nytimes.com/2008/01/03/outsourced-wombs/.
95. Satz, *Why Some Things Should Not Be for Sale*, 124.
96. Anderson, "Why Commercial Surrogate Motherhood Unethically Commodifies Women and Children," *Health Care Analysis* 8 (2000): 19–26, at 25.

97. Anderson, "Is Women's Labor a Commodity?," 88.
98. Hugh LaFollette, "Licensing Parents," *Philosophy and Public Affairs* 9 (1980): 182–197.
99. For extended discussion of state action to prevent conception, see Harry Adams, *Justice for Children: Autonomy Development and the State* (Albany: SUNY Press, 2008), 117–153. Adams ends up supporting compulsory contraception in principle in an ideally just state, but opposing it in fact in the United States, given this nation's recent if not ongoing history of racism, sexism, and classism.
100. Rebecca Dresser, "Screen the Parents," in "The Baby Market," http:// roomfordebate.blogs.nytimes.com/2009/12/29/the-baby-market/. Compare Satz, *Why Some Things Should Not Be for Sale*, 127: "It is a good question as to why decisions involved in assisted reproductive technology are assumed to be a highly private matter, despite the involvement of third parties."

NOTES TO CHAPTER 5

1. Kenneth Henley, "The Authority to Educate," in *Having Children*, eds. O'Neill and Ruddick, 254–264, at 262. For reasons to credit the claim that Henley appears to doubt, see John A. Hostetler, "The Amish Way of Life Is at Stake (1966)," in *Writing the Amish: The Worlds of John A. Hostetler*, ed. David L. Weaver-Zercher (University Park: The Pennsylvania State University Press, 2004), 233–235; Donald B. Kraybill, *The Riddle of Amish Culture* (Baltimore: The Johns Hopkins University Press, 1989), 130–134; and Thomas J. Meyers, "Education and Schooling," in *The Amish and the State*, ed. Donald B. Kraybill (Baltimore: The Johns Hopkins University Press, 1993), 86–106, at 102–104. For an account of the diversity of Amish educational practices, see Karen M. Johnson-Weiner, *Train Up a Child: Old Order and Amish and Mennonite Schools* (Baltimore: The Johns Hopkins University Press, 2007), especially 229–245.
2. Feinberg, "The Child's Right to an Open Future," in *Freedom and Fulfillment*, 76–97, at 86. It should be noted that Feinberg nevertheless does not contend that the decision in *Yoder* was "mistaken." As he writes on the same page, given the fact that "[t]he difference between a mere eight years of elementary education and a mere ten years of mostly elementary education seems so trivial in the technologically complex modern world . . ., [i]t is plausible therefore to argue that what is gained for the educable fourteen-year-old Amish youth by guaranteeing him another two years of school is more than counterbalanced by the corrosive effect on the religious bonds of the Amish community."
3. Robert Filmer, *Patriarcha*, in *Patriarcha and Other Writings*, ed. Johann P. Immerville (Cambridge: Cambridge University Press, 1991), chapter 2, §4, pp. 18–19. It seems that Filmer took this story from Jean Bodin's *Six livres de la république*, bk. 1, ch. 4; in any event, the story is likely apocryphal.
4. See further on *patria potestas* Boswell, *The Kindness of Strangers*, 58–59.
5. John Rawls, *A Theory of Justice* (Cambridge, MA: Harvard University Press, 1971), 31. See also Rawls's *Political Liberalism* (New York: Columbia University Press, 1996), 173–211, especially 174: "In justice as fairness the priority of right means that the principles of political justice impose limits on permissible ways of life; and hence the claims citizens make to pursue ends that transgress those limits have no weight."

6. For an argument casting doubt on the enhancement project on scientific grounds, see, however, Philip M. Rosoff, "The Myth of Genetic Enhancement," *Theoretical Medicine and Bioethics* 33 (2012): 163–178.
7. Jean-Jacques Rousseau, *Du contrat social ou Principes du droit politique* (Paris: Garnier Frères, 1962), bk. 1, ch. 1, p. 236. As translators often note, "L'homme est né libre" may be rendered either, "Man was born free," or "Man is born free."
8. Thomas Hobbes, *Leviathan*, ed. Edwin Curley (Indianapolis, IN: Hackett, 1994), pt. 2, ch. 20, §§4–5, pp. 128–130.
9. Locke, *Second Treatise of Government*, §55, p. 304 (equality), §61, p. 308 (freedom).
10. Jeffrey Morgan, "Children's Rights and the Parental Authority to Instill a Specific Value System," *Essays in Philosophy* 7/1 (2006): n.p. (accessed online at http://commons.pacificu.edu/cgi/viewcontent.cgi?article=1226& context=eip). Morgan does not define what he means by indoctrination, the fighting word here.
11. See Michael Walzer, *Exodus and Revolution* (New York: Basic Books, 1985), 86: "In Spain, in the years before the Expulsion, when many Jews 'turned away' from the covenant . . ., the obvious question was asked: 'Who gave the generation of the wilderness which stood at the foot of Mount Sinai the power of obligating all those who would arise after them?'"
12. Locke, *The First Treatise of Government*, in *Two Treatises*, §51, p. 177.
13. Hobbes, *Leviathan*, pt. 2, ch. 20, §4, p.128. He writes in §5, p. 129 that "if [the mother] nourish [the infant], it oweth its life to the mother, and is therefore obliged to obey her rather than any other, and by consequence the dominion over it is hers."
14. See Blustein, *Parents and Children: The Ethics of the Family* (New York: Oxford University Press, 1982), 107–108.
15. Amy Gutmann, "Children, Paternalism, and Education: A Liberal Argument," *Philosophy and Public Affairs* 9 (1980): 338–358, at 339.
16. Locke, *Second Treatise*, §58, p. 306.
17. Ibid., §67, p. 312.
18. Robert Noggle, "Special Agents: Children's Autonomy and Parental Authority," in *The Moral and Political Status of Children*, eds. David Archard and Colin Macleod (Oxford: Oxford University Press, 2002), 97–117, at 101.
19. Blustein presents and defends the Lockean "thesis of the priority of parental duties to parental rights" in his *Parents and Children*, 111–114. As Blustein notes, it follows from the claim that parental duties take priority over parental rights that "[p]arents . . . are entitled to take their own interests into account *in* discharging their duties," but "they may not pursue their own interests instead of discharging their duties" (114).
20. See for discussion Archard, "The Obligations and Responsibilities of Parenthood," 106–109. I agree with him that "rights and obligations have different kinds of ground," and that one may incur at least some measure of parental obligations to a child without gaining any parental rights (107), as ought to be the case with male rapists. See on this last point Shauna R. Prewitt, "Giving Birth to a 'Rapist's Child': A Discussion and Analysis of the Limited Legal Protections Afforded to Women Who Become Mothers through Rape," *Georgetown Law Journal* 98 (2010): 827–862. Prewitt notes that "few states have passed special laws to aid the large number of raped women who choose to raise their rape-conceived children. Without such laws, a man who fathers a child

through rape has the same custody and visitation privileges regarding that child as does the father of a child not conceived through rape" (829). Another complicated question concerns whether an unwed father has the right to veto an adoption decision of an unwed mother, one of the questions raised in the notorious case of *Baby Girl Clausen* (199 Mich. App. 10, 501 N.W.2d 193 [1993]). See for discussion Shanley, "Fathers' Rights, Mothers' Wrongs?," 88–96.

21. Samantha Brennan and Robert Noggle, "The Moral Status of Children: Children's Rights, Parents' Rights, and Family Justice," *Social Theory and Practice* 23 (1997): 1–26, at 11. This conception of the parent-child relationship is nonetheless a relatively recent innovation in the law. As Robert K. Vischer notes, "Until the late nineteenth century, the legal system treated children wholly as the property of parents, even in cases of extreme abuse and neglect. The first successfully prosecuted child-abuse case did not occur [in the United States] until 1874—and given the lack of a relevant statute, had to be brought under laws prohibiting animal cruelty." This was the case of Mary Ellen Wilson. See Vischer, "All in the Family: When Should the State Intervene?" *Commonweal*, March 23, 2007, 8.

22. See Noggle, "Special Agents," 98. As he notes, the physician or the lawyer in a fiduciary relationship "does not have authority over the patient or client in the way that the parent is typically thought to have (at least limited) authority over the child."

23. Ibid., 106.

24. Gutmann, "Children, Paternalism, and Education," 339. See also Noggle, "Special Agents," 107.

25. Rawls, *A Theory of Justice*, 249 (paternalism) and 62 (primary goods). See also 209 for a preliminary articulation of "the principle of paternalism."

26. Gutmann, "Children, Paternalism, and Education," 341.

27. Henley, "The Authority to Educate," 256.

28. Feinberg, "The Child's Right to an Open Future," 78, 80. Feinberg has been rightly criticized for saying that a child's opportunities must be "maximized." (See also "The Child's Right to an Open Future," 84: "[Education] should send [a child] out into the adult world with as many opportunities as possible, thus maximizing his chances for self-fulfillment.") How, it has been asked, should these opportunities be quantified; is not the *variety* of the options, which is surely more important than the sheer number anyway, a matter of perspective; and do not some opportunities require such concentration that others must be excluded? See Claudia Mills, "The Child's Right to an Open Future?" *Journal of Social Philosophy* 34 (2003): 499–509, at 500–503, who makes the nice observation that "from the point of view of the Amish farmer," the career options that Feinberg complains are closed to Amish children—engineer, research scientist, lawyer, business executive—"have little variety among them: They are all ways of living in the world, pursuing money, prestige, and professional satisfaction. . . ." See for similar criticisms Richard J. Arneson and Ian Shapiro, "Democratic Autonomy and Religious Freedom: A Critique of *Wisconsin v. Yoder*," in *Political Order: Nomos XXXVIII*, eds. Ian Shapiro and Russell Hardin (New York: New York University Press, 1996), 365–411, at 391–393. In criticizing *Yoder*, Arneson and Shapiro nonetheless make claims similar to Feinberg's. For example, they write that, "[a]s a fiduciary, the parent is bound to preserve the child's own future religious freedom" (384)—in a word, though not Arneson and Shapiro's, to keep it "open."

29. Nicholas Agar, *Liberal Eugenics: In Defence of Human Enhancement* (Oxford: Blackwell, 2004), 124. Agar holds that educating children in such a way would be wrong.

30. See Eamonn Callan, "Autonomy, Child-Rearing, and Good Lives," in *The Moral and Political Status of Children*, 118–141, at 121; and Archard, "Children, Multiculturalism, and Education," in *The Moral and Political Status of Children*, 142–159, at 156. There are, to be sure, more elaborate conceptions of autonomy than found in the children's rights literature. For example, David DeGrazia proposes that "A autonomously performs intentional action X if and only if (1) A does X because she prefers to do X, (2) A has this preference because she (at least dispositionally) identifies with and prefers to do X, and (3) this identification has not resulted primarily from influences that A would, on careful reflection, consider alienating." See DeGrazia's *Human Identity and Bioethics* (Cambridge: Cambridge University Press, 2005), 102.

31. Gutmann, "Children, Paternalism, and Education," 341. Compare Rawls, *Political Liberalism*, 180–181.

32. Ibid., 347.

33. Ibid., 341, 342.

34. Ibid., 348, 349. See, in support of the claim that "the fact that *some* choice is good doesn't necessarily mean that *more* choice is better," Barry Schwartz, *The Paradox of Choice: Why More Is Less* (New York: HarperCollins, 2004), 3.

35. Ibid., 349.

36. Gutmann never says just what she takes a society to be, but she apparently holds that Amish society does not qualify—though social scientists who have studied the Amish do not show any such qualms, and the dictionary does not give any reason to be uneasy. (According to the OED, a society may be defined as "[t]he aggregate of persons living together in a more or less ordered community," or "[a] number of persons associated together by some common interest or purpose, united by a common vow, holding the same belief or opinion, following the same trade or profession, etc.") Gutmann has somewhat more to say about "the unusually separatist existence of the Old Amish Order" in her article "Civic Education and Diversity," *Ethics* 10 (1995): 557–579, at 568–570. In particular, she notes that the Court's decision in *Yoder* may be defended given "the exceptionalism of the Amish among religious groups in the United States." Yet, though she acknowledges that this defense is "reasonable," she neither retracts nor modifies her criticism of the decision.

37. Compare Rawls, *Political Liberalism*, 199, who likewise speaks of "society" monolithically.

38. Kraybill, *The Riddle of Amish Culture*, 252, 140. Kraybill comes to this judgment despite the rather sensationalized phenomenon of "Rumspringa" or "wilding" among Amish teens. According to Kraybill, "Flings with worldliness gives Amish youth the impression that they have a choice regarding church membership," but for most "the perceived choice is partially an illusion" (140).

39. See Harry Brighouse, "Civic Education and Liberal Legitimacy," *Ethics* 108 (1998): 719–745, at 743, who advocates "autonomy-facilitating education" for its potential to "*mitigate* the tendency of former believers to bitterness, so that when people abandon their parents' way of life for another they do so not irrationally and with resentment, but with a cool appreciation of the goods and bads of both." See also Callan, "Autonomy, Child-Rearing, and Good Lives," 140, n. 7, who reports a criticism raised by Archard of the

kind of religious upbringing the philosopher Nicholas Wolterstorff writes he had: one that "implanted in [him] an interpretation of reality—a fundamental hermeneutic" that sank so deep into his consciousness "that nothing thereafter, short of senility," could remove it (Wolterstorff quoted by Callan, "Autonomy, Child-Rearing, and Good Lives," 128). According to Archard, as Callan paraphrases him, this kind of upbringing could "block autonomous choice by making the emotional costs of choosing against the values of one's upbringing prohibitively high."

40. Michael J. Sandel, "The Procedural Republic and the Unencumbered Self," in *Public Philosophy: Essays on Morality in Politics* (Cambridge, MA: Harvard University Press, 2005), 167.

41. Mark Twain, *Adventures of Huckleberry Finn*, in *Huck Finn; Pudd'nhead Wilson; No. 44, The Mysterious Stranger; and Other Writings* (New York: Library of America, 2000), ch. 5, p. 28: "'And looky here—you drop that school, you hear? I'll learn people to bring up a boy to put on airs over his own father and let on to be better'n what *he* is. You lemme catch you fooling around that school again, you hear? Your mother couldn't read, and she couldn't write, nuther, before she died. None of the family couldn't, before *they* died. *I* can't; and here you're a-swelling yourself up like this. I ain't the man to stand it—you hear?'"

42. Gutmann, "Children, Paternalism, and Education," 348.

43. 406 U.S. 205, 238 (1972).

44. Gutmann, "Children, Paternalism, and Education," 348, n. 14.

45. 406 U.S. 205, 222 (1972). Compare the majority opinion of Sixth Circuit Chief Judge Pierce Lively in *Mozert v. Hawkins County*, 827 F.2d 1058, 1067 (1987), another case that is sometimes discussed in the children's rights literature: "The parents in Yoder were required to send their children to some school that prepared them for life in the outside world, or face official sanctions. The parents in the present case want their children to acquire all the skills required to live in modern society"—thus leading to his rejection of *Yoder* as a relevant precedent. See, however, for critical discussion of the *Mozert* court's reasoning Shelley Burtt, "Religious Parents, Secular Schools: A Liberal Defense of an Illiberal Education," *The Review of Politics* 56 (1994): 51–70, especially 56–59 and 61–67.

46. Feinberg, "The Child's Right to an Open Future," 84.

47. Remarkably, Feinberg claims that his view of the goal of education is neutral between the two alternatives that Burger lays out. See ibid.

48. Ibid., 82.

49. Compare Brian Barry, *Culture and Equality: An Egalitarian Critique of Multiculturalism* (Cambridge: Polity, 2001), 211, who considers "three possible answers" to the question of the interest of the child in education: (1) "to be able to function successfully in the world into which [he or she] is going to grow up"; (2) "for the sake of living well"; and (3) to become autonomous.

50. Burtt, "Reproductive Responsibilities," 190.

51. Burtt, "In Defense of *Yoder*: Parental Authority and the Public Schools," in *Political Order*, 412–437, at 429.

52. Buchanan, Brock, Daniels, and Wikler, *From Chance to Choice*, 170.

53. Again compare Barry, *Culture and Equality*, 217, who writes that the "key" question is, "if education should prepare children to get by in the world they will grow up into, how is that world to be defined?" So far as I can tell, though, he does not answer this question. He also does not say that we should consider the goodness of life within the "world" in question. See also Johnson-Weiner, *Train Up a Child*, 233: "Which world? is

the question that guides Old Order communities as they establish private schools that, from the most conservative to the most progressive, reflect and reinforce the values of the church-community."

54. See again Schwartz, *The Paradox of Choice*, 99: "though modern Americans have more choice than any group of people ever has before, and thus, presumably, more freedom and autonomy, we don't seem to be benefiting from [this increased choice] psychologically." (The title of the chapter from which this quotation is taken is "Choice and Happiness.") Interestingly, Schwartz contrasts in this regard "mainstream America" with "Amish society, where expectations about individual control and autonomy are very different"—and the incidence of depression, among the Amish in Lancaster County in any event, "is less than 20 percent of the national rate" (212).

55. It is worth noting on this point that Arneson and Shapiro's principal criticism of *Yoder* is that an "adequate conception of democratic citizenship compels the conclusion that compulsory high school attendance is a reasonable state requirement for the purpose of preparing youth for the role of citizen." For they claim that in order "[t]o be able to participate competently in democratic decision-making, voters should have an adequate knowledge of contemporary science in its bearing on public policy issues, an understanding of modern world history and particularly the history of democratic institutions and the culture of their own society, and critical thinking skills that include the ability to represent the situation of others in imagination, to intuit their experience, and sympathetically to analyze and assess their attitudes, principles, and policy arguments." See "Democratic Autonomy and Religious Freedom," 375, 376. As Burtt notes, however, "There are a number of difficulties with a critique of *Yoder* along these lines." To begin with, this standard of responsible citizenship seems to demand far more than high school education, and certainly far more than the education offered in most public high schools in the contemporary United States. More fundamentally, Burtt also draws attention to the odd and perhaps even troubling "assumption embedded not only in Arneson and Shapiro's work but in most recent philosophical considerations of critical rationality," namely, "that to reason from the basis of God's word as reflected in Scripture," as the Amish do, "is somehow to abandon the exercise of critical rationality" and to sacrifice all the "critical thinking skills" that Arneson and Shapiro consider necessary to responsible citizenship. See "In Defense of *Yoder*," 415–416.

56. See Burtt, "In Defense of *Yoder*," 420–421.

57. See 406 U.S. 205, 225 (1972): "The Amish alternative to formal secondary school education has enabled them to function effectively in their day-to-day life under self-imposed limitations on relations with the world, and to survive and prosper in contemporary society as a separate, sharply identifiable and highly self-sufficient community for more than 200 years in this country." On this "Amish alternative," see further Hostetler, "Old Order Amish Child Rearing and School Practices: A Summary Report (1970)," in *Writing the Amish*, 236–250.

58. See 406 U.S. 205, 224–225 (1972): "There is nothing in this record to suggest that the Amish qualities of reliability, self-reliance, and dedication to work would fail to find ready markets in today's [greater American] society. Absent some contrary evidence supporting the State's position, we are unwilling to assume that persons possessing such valuable vocational skills and habits are doomed to become burdens on [greater American] society should they determine to leave the Amish faith. . . ." See also 234:

"The record strongly indicates that accommodating the religious objections of the Amish by forgoing one, or at most two, additional years of compulsory education will not impair the physical or mental health of the child, or result in an inability to be self-supporting or to discharge the duties and responsibilities of citizenship. . . ." By the way, Burtt's reading of the Opinion of the Court in *Yoder* is much more critical than mine: she defends the outcome, but not much of the reasoning.

59. William A. Galston, "Two Concepts of Liberalism," *Ethics* 105 (1995): 516–534, at 521.

60. Ibid., 523. Barry has criticized "Galston's notion of 'Reformation liberalism' [as] an oxymoron," pointing out that, as a matter of historical record, neither Luther, Calvin, nor the Anabaptists supported the separation of church and state. See *Culture and Equality*, 177. I take it, however, that Galston's point in looking back to the Reformation is that liberalism developed as a response to the conflicts that characterized this era, not that the Reformers themselves were liberals or even proto-liberals. (Rawls tells a similar story in the introduction to his *Political Liberalism*, xxv–xxvi.) Galston himself answers the common charge that "diversity requires tolerance, and tolerance cannot be sustained without critical reflection on ways of life, including one's own." In his words, "The heart of tolerance a liberal society needs is the refusal to use state power to impose one's own way of life on others," and there is no necessary incompatibility between such refusal and an unreflective commitment to a particular way of life. See "Two Concepts of Liberalism," 524.

61. Kraybill, *The Riddle of Amish Culture*, 252–253. Compare Burtt, "In Defense of *Yoder*," 425, who claims that Arneson and Shapiro work with "too narrow an account of children's interests, one which excludes from consideration not only the needs of the children as moral and spiritual beings, but their interests as members of distinct cultural communities."

62. Callan, "Autonomy, Child-Rearing, and Good Lives," 135.

63. See for further discussion and citations my "Rethinking 'Liberal Eugenics': Reflections and Questions on Habermas on Bioethics," *Hastings Center Report* 35/6 (2005): 31–42, especially 32–34.

64. Buchanan et al., *From Chance to Choice*, 171.

65. Agar, "Liberal Eugenics," *Public Affairs Quarterly* 12 (1998): 135–155, at 145.

66. Ibid., 150. Agar's formulation parallels Rawls's two principles of justice; see *A Theory of Justice*, 302–303. A maximin rule, as Rawls states, "tells us to rank alternatives by their worst possible outcomes: we are to adopt the alternative the worst outcome of which is superior to the outcome of the others." See *A Theory of Justice*, 152–153.

67. Ibid. See also Buchanan et al., *From Chance to Choice*, 167–168, who propose that we recognize "natural primary goods" analogous to Rawls's "social primary goods," namely, "'general purpose' means useful or valuable in carrying out nearly any plan of life." (See *A Theory of Justice*, 92.)

68. In his recent book of the same title as his article, *Liberal Eugenics*, Agar appeals to the concept of "real freedom," borrowed from Amartya Sen and Martha Nussbaum, for light in how to regulate enhancement technologies. In Agar's use, a person's real freedom refers to "her capacity to choose one way of life in preference to others." A person has greater or lesser real freedom depending on the range of "alternative functionings"—that is, "the various things a person may value doing or being"— open to her. In order to respect a prospective child's autonomy, parents

must "not, in the pursuit of their eugenic visions, *reduce* their children's real freedom, or have children with *less* real freedom than those they would otherwise have had." An enhancement reduces real freedom "if it makes unlikely a successful life founded on values that oppose those of the enhancers." As an example, Agar cites the case of an Amish child who "has no realistic prospect of pursuing a lifestyle radically opposed to Amish values." According to him, such an upbringing "is likely to infringe autonomy" (that is, self-determination) and so would be prohibited by the precept that real freedom must not be reduced. See *Liberal Eugenics*, 104, 124. What remains critical, despite the new vocabulary, is that a child's parents keep his or her future "open."

69. Agar, "Liberal Eugenics," 179.
70. Ibid., 181.
71. Ibid., 176.
72. Agar, "Designing Babies: Morally Permissible Ways to Modify the Human Genome," *Bioethics* 9 (1995): 1–15, at 14.
73. See again Rosoff, "The Myth of Genetic Enhancement," 170–173.
74. Robertson, *Children of Choice*, 165–166.
75. Compare (or contrast) Leon Kass on what we might expect of parents who decided "to clone a Rubinstein"; see his "Making Babies: The New Biology and the 'Old' Morality," in *Toward a More Natural Science: Biology and Human Affairs* (New York: The Free Press, 1985), 43–79, at 68–69.
76. On whether the obligation in question is "perfect" or "imperfect," I am reluctant to say that a child has a *right* to be loved. Imagine a child seeking a lawyer to press charges against his or her parents for not loving him or her. Perhaps the hint of comedy here lies in the idea of a child entering a law office with this intent, or in the suggestion that an obligation to love is legally enforceable, as if the threat of some jail time might make parents shape up; but it also seems comic to imagine a child insisting on his or her right to be loved, all threat of legal action aside. In other words, there is something "off" about the complaint that his or her right to be loved has been violated. By contrast, the accusation, "You don't love me," with the implication that the parent ought to do so, has no comic overtones at all. In brief, whereas the claim that a parent has an obligation to love his or her child appears to make perfect sense, the claim that a child has a right to be loved seems to stretch the language of rights beyond its limit, or at least its usefulness. I think it makes better sense, then, to categorize the obligation in question as an *imperfect* obligation, using this term in contrast to a perfect obligation to mark the distinction between obligations with counterpart rights (namely, perfect obligations) and obligations without counterpart rights (namely, imperfect obligations). Yet more precisely, the obligation in question appears to be a *special* imperfect obligation, as it comes with being a parent, and it is possible to specify to whom the obligation is owed, namely, the parent's child or children. The obligation is also "imperfect" in the sense that the ways in which it is to be discharged will vary quite widely according to the circumstances of culture. That the obligation is apparently "imperfect" does not, however, lessen its importance; only a fascination with the category of rights might make us think so. Contrast Liao, "The Right of Children to Be Loved," 422, claiming (1) that "[h]uman beings have rights to those conditions that are primary essential for a good life"; (2) that "[b]eing loved is primary essential for children to have a good life" as human beings (for which he provides much important documentation); and so (3) that,

"[t]herefore, children have a right to be loved" (422). I acknowledge that it might be claimed that a child has either a so-called imperfect right to be loved (a claim of *humanity* against others), or what the Protestant natural lawyers called an oeconomical right (not a private or natural right that one possesses qua human being, but a right that one possesses qua child of identifiable parents), but these categories have fallen into desuetude.

77. I take these examples from Buchanan, "Enhancement and the Ethics of Development," *Kennedy Institute of Ethics Journal* 18/1 (2008): 1–34, at 8.

78. Brock, "Is Selection of Children Wrong?" in *Human Enhancement*, eds. Julian Savulescu and Nick Bostrom (Oxford: Oxford University Press, 2009), 251–276, at 269. See also 270, and Frances Kamm, "What Is and Is Not Wrong with Enhancement," in *Human Enhancement*, 91–130, at 110: "much of ordinary good parenting consists of what might be called enhancement."

79. See for critical discussion, however, Colin Macleod, "Parental Responsibilities in an Unjust World," in *Procreation and Parenthood*, 128–150.

80. Brock, "Is Selection of Children Wrong?," 269.

81. Ibid., 270.

82. See Sandel, "The Case against Perfection: What's Wrong with Designer Children, Bionic Athletes, and Genetic Engineering," in *The Atlantic Monthly*, April 2004, 51–54, 56–60, 62, especially 56–58; reprinted in *Human Enhancement*, 71–89, especially 79–82; and incorporated into *The Case against Perfection* (Cambridge, MA: Harvard University Press, 2007), especially 45ff.

83. See Kamm, "What Is and Is Not Wrong with Enhancement," 113. See also 117: "searching for more than the basics does not by itself imply that if one could not achieve those enhancements, one would not still happily have a child who had only the basics, and love the particular person she is. . . ."

84. Ibid., 117.

85. See for a subtle and illuminating discussion, however, Erik Malmqvist, "Reprogenetics and the 'Parents Have Always Done It' Argument," *Hastings Center Report* 41/1 (2011): 43–49.

86. Schwartz, *The Paradox of Choice*, 191.

87. Kamm, "What Is and Is Not Wrong with Enhancement," 117.

88. Schwartz, *The Paradox of Choice*, 183.

89. See for discussion of "when men don't want to father" Susan S. Lang, *Women without Children: The Reasons, the Rewards, the Regrets* (New York: Pharos Books, 1991), 108–109.

90. Brock, "Is Selection of Children Wrong?," 271.

91. Barbara Katz Rothman, *The Tentative Pregnancy: Amniocentesis and the Sexual Politics of Motherhood* (New York: W. W. Norton, 1993), 7.

92. I thank a referee for this suggestion.

93. Rothman, *The Tentative Pregnancy*, 7. See also 87, 101–103. Compare Burtt, "Which Babies? Dilemmas of Genetic Testing," *Tikkun* 16/1 (2001): 45–47.

94. Sandel, "The Case against Perfection," 58 (reprint, 81; *The Case against Perfection*, 52).

95. See Winnicott, *The Maturational Processes and the Facilitating Environment*, 71, 147, on identification; and 96, 148, on adaptation.

96. Mills, "The Child's Right to an Open Future?," 505, 507. To be accurate, Mills writes that "[t]he wrong of overly directive child rearing is less a sin against autonomy than a sin against love." I think, however, that it is more

correct to say that the wrong in question is *as much* a sin against love as it is against autonomy.

97. Ibid., 505. It should be noted, however, that Amish parents do not "shun" children who decide against baptism into the community. Instead, shunning is reserved for persons who seek baptism but then fall away from the faith.

98. Kant, *Kritik der reinen Vernunft*, ed. Raymund Schmidt, 3rd ed. (Hamburg: Felix Meiner, 1990), 599, A634/B662–A635/B663; *Critique of Pure Reason*, trans. Norman Kemp Smith (New York: St. Martin's Press, 1929), 527.

99. Kant, "Mutmaßlicher Angfang der Menschengeschichte," in vol. 4 of his *Werke, Schriften von 1783–1788*, eds. Artur Buchenau and Ernst Cassirer (Berlin: Bruno Cassirer, 1922), 327; "Speculative Beginning of Human History," in *Perpetual Peace and Other Essays*, trans. Ted Humphrey (Indianapolis, IN: Hackett, 1983), 49.

100. See Wilkinson, *Choosing Tomorrow's Children*, 31.

102. Compare Buchanan, "Enhancement and the Ethics of Development," 18.

102. Here is another worry. It may be argued that parents have an obligation not only to preserve a child's "open future," but to maximize this openness through the use of genetic enhancements. Julian Savulescu's oft-cited "Procreative Beneficence: Why We Should Select the Best Children," *Bioethics* 15 (2001): 413–426, moves in this direction, as does John Harris's *Enhancing Evolution: The Ethical Case for Making Better People*. As the flipside of a consequentialist argument that parents have a moral obligation to reduce suffering is that parents have a moral obligation to increase happiness, the surprising upshot is that we are morally obliged to pursue a project of human enhancement. I agree with Robert Sparrow that this argument resurrects the danger of eugenics. See his "A Not-So-New Eugenics: Harris and Savulescu on Human Enhancement," *Hastings Center Report* 41/1 (2011): 32–42.

103. I thank a referee for the formulation of this position.

104. Wilkinson, *Choosing Tomorrow's Children*, 29.

105. Ibid., 30.

106. Schwartz, *The Paradox of Choice*, 96, 77. Unfortunately, at present, there are no studies to support or for that matter refute this suggestion (Barry Schwartz, personal communication, December 28, 2012, cited with his permission).

NOTES TO CHAPTER 6

1. LaFollette, "Licensing Parents," 193.

2. Ibid., 187: "a person has a right to rear children if he meets certain minimal standards of child rearing."

3. Ibid., 196.

4. Locke, *Second Treatise*, §27, p. 288. See for discussion Nozick, *Anarchy, State, Utopia*, 287–289, commenting on the conjunction of Locke's theories of property and parenthood.

5. As Ferdinand Schoeman notes, citing a U.S. national survey, "establishing such relationships tends to be the primary reason adults in our culture give for wanting and having children." See Schoeman, "Rights of Children, Rights of Parents, and the Moral Basis of the Family," 8.

6. Compare ibid., 14–16. To quote this last page, "while the state is quite limited in its ability to promote relationships, it can do much to destroy them."

7. LaFollette, "Licensing Parents," 190.
8. Schrag, "Justice and the Family," 193.
9. It might also be objected that my ideal of the parent-child relationship is all too Western and modern, or in a word "culture-bound." I am reminded here of an objection that Robert Nozick put to Elizabeth Anderson. Against her claim that a child ought to be loved by his or her parents and not valued as a mere "use-object" or commodity that may properly be bought and sold, he asked (in Anderson's words), "Do not parents in the Third World, who rely on children to provide for the family subsistence, regard their children as economic goods?" We might also think of parents who callously sell daughters into prostitution. Anderson's twofold response to this objection seems to me correct. First, children who promote the livelihood of their family "need not be treated in accordance with market norms" (meaning as mere commodities), and what's more they usually remain part of a family and often benefit from parental love. Second, insofar as children are treated as mere commodities (take daughters sold into prostitution), "this treatment is deplorable wherever it takes place"—full stop. See Anderson, "Is Women's Labor a Commodity?," 77, n. 10.
10. Blustein, "Doing the Best for One's Child," 200.
11. It should also be noted that I do not address responsibilities to children beyond our borders. A fuller discussion would have to engage Colin Macleod's "Parental Responsibilities in an Unjust World," in *Procreation and Parenthood*, 128–150. Richard W. Miller's *Globalizing Justice: The Ethics of Poverty and Power* (Oxford: Oxford University Press, 2010), 13–21, provides a place to begin.
12. See, for example, Rolf George, "Who Should Bear the Cost of Children?" *Public Affairs Quarterly* 1 (1987): 1–42; and "On the External Benefits of Children," in *Kindred Matters: Rethinking the Philosophy of the Family*, eds. Diana Tietjens Meyers, Kenneth Kipnis, and Cornelius F. Murphy, Jr. (Ithaca, NY: Cornell University Press, 1993), 209–217.
13. Plato, *The Republic*, trans. Allan Bloom, 2nd ed. (New York: Basic Books, 1968), book 5, 463c, p. 143.
14. Ibid., 464c–d, p. 144.
15. Ibid., 464d.
16. Zelizer, *Pricing the Priceless Child*, xiii.
17. Rawls, *A Theory of Justice*, 302.
18. Ibid., 303. See also 43, where Rawls states that he will propose "ranking the principle of equal liberty prior to the principle regulating economic and social inequalities."
19. Ibid., 74.
20. James Fishkin, *Justice, Equal Opportunity, and the Family* (New Haven, CT: Yale University Press, 1983), 52, citing data and studies as well.
21. Rawls, *A Theory of Justice*, 511.
22. Ibid., 511–512.
23. Ibid, 43–44.
24. Schrag, "Justice and the Family," 197. I have followed Schrag in laying out my criticisms of Rawls's theory on this point. A possible defense, however, should be noted. Rawls allows the parties to the original position to have a basic knowledge of history, psychology, and sociology. Though Rawls does not himself defend the family on these grounds, perhaps it could be claimed that the parties to the original position would retain the family, and not even entertain its abolition, in the light of what they know about human beings. I thank Daniel Thero for this suggestion.
25. Fishkin, *Justice, Equal Opportunity, and the Family*, 132.

26. Ibid., 61. See also 55.
27. Ibid., 65.
28. Schrag, "Justice and the Family," 195. I take this characterization of a maximin strategy from Rawls, *A Theory of Justice*, 153.
29. Schrag, "Justice and the Family," 195.
30. Rawls, *A Theory of Justice*, 3.
31. See Schrag, "Justice and the Family," 197.
32. Ibid., 203.
33. Ibid.
34. Kolodny, "Which Relationships Justify Partiality?," 68.
35. See Fishkin, *Justice, Equal Opportunity, and the Family*, 54–55.
36. Ibid., 154.
37. Ibid.
38. See Williams, "Ethical Consistency," in *Problems of the Self*, 166–186, at 172.
39. Ibid., 183.
40. Compare a conflict between two desires: here too there is the possibility of struggle without the winner diminishing the loser. By way of example, the young Augustine sorely desired chastity and continence—only, he told his God at one point, just not yet. See Augustine, *Confessions*, ed. James J. O'Donnell (Oxford: Oxford University Press, 1992), vol. 1, book 8, 7(17), p. 96: "'*da mihi castitatem et continentiam, sed noli modo.*'"
41. See for discussion David Brooks, "When Families Fail," *New York Times*, February 14, 2013, sec. A, advocating expansion of early education projects, as President Obama proposed in his 2013 State of the Union address.
42. See by way of example Michael Funke, "Fostering Independence: State Responsibility for Emancipated Youth" (unpublished paper), which documents, among other grim statistics, the high rates of homelessness of emancipated foster youth and advocates the expansion of Independent Living Programs as means to help these youth develop into autonomous adults.
43. See the important book by Matthew A. Crenson, *Building the Invisible Orphanage: A Prehistory of the American Welfare System* (Cambridge, MA: Harvard University Press, 1998).
44. See, to begin with, the Children's Defense Fund's report *The State of America's Children 2011*, available online through the CDF. The news is not good. As the report states, "CDF's *State of America's Children 2011* paints a devastating portrait of childhood across the country. With unemployment, housing foreclosures and hunger still at historically high levels, children's well-being is in great jeopardy" (ix). See further David Brooks, "The Opportunity Gap," *New York Times*, July 10, 2012, sec. A, on research documenting the fast growing inequality of opportunities among children of the affluent and the poor.
45. See again, as a starting point for reflection, Miller, *Globalizing Justice*, 13–21, who defends the "prerogative to express one's valuing of a parental relationship to one's child in special concern for her, so long as greater sensitivity to others' neediness as such would impose a significant risk of worsening her life" (21).

Bibliography

Adams, Harry. *Justice for Children: Autonomy Development and the State*. Albany, N.Y.: SUNY Press, 2008.

Agar, Nicholas. "Designing Babies: Morally Permissible Ways to Modify the Human Genome." *Bioethics* 9 (1995): 1–15.

———. "Liberal Eugenics." *Public Affairs Quarterly* 12 (1998): 135–155.

———. *Liberal Eugenics: In Defence of Human Enhancement*. Oxford: Blackwell, 2004.

Alstott, Anne L. *No Exit: What Parents Owe Their Children and What Society Owes Parents*. Oxford: Oxford University Press, 2004.

Alter, Robert, trans. *The David Story*. New York: W.W. Norton, 1999.

———, trans. *The Five Books of Moses*. New York: W.W. Norton, 2004.

Anderson, Elizabeth S. "Is Women's Labor a Commodity?" *Philosophy and Public Affairs* 19 (1990): 71–92.

———. "Why Commercial Surrogate Motherhood Unethically Commodifies Women and Children." *Health Care Analysis* 8 (2000): 19–26.

Andrews, Lori B. "Surrogate Motherhood: The Challenge for Feminists." *Journal of Law, Medicine, and Health Care* 16 (1988): 72–80.

Archard, David. "Children, Multiculturalism, and Education." In *The Moral and Political Status of Children*, edited by David Archard and Colin Macleod, 142–159. Oxford: Oxford University Press, 2002.

———. *Children: Rights and Childhood*. London: Routledge, 1993.

———. "The Obligations and Responsibilities of Parenthood." In *Procreation and Parenthood: The Ethics of Bearing and Rearing Children*, edited by David Archard and David Benatar, 103–127. Oxford: Oxford University Press, 2010.

Arneson, Richard J. "Commodification and Commercial Surrogacy." *Philosophy and Public Affairs* 21 (1992): 132–164.

Arneson, Richard J., and Ian Shapiro. "Democratic Autonomy and Religious Freedom: A Critique of *Wisconsin v. Yoder*." In *Political Order: Nomos XXXVIII*, edited by Ian Shapiro and Russell Hardin, 365–411. New York: New York University Press, 1996.

Atighetchi, Dariusch. *Islamic Bioethics: Problems and Perspectives*. Dordrecht: Springer, 2007.

Augustine. *Confessions*. Edited by James J. O'Donnell. Vol. 1. Oxford: Oxford University Press, 1992.

Austin, Michael W. *Conceptions of Parenthood: Ethics and the Family*. Aldershot: Ashgate, 2007.

Barad, David H., and Brian L. Cohen. "Oocyte Donation Program at Montefiore Medical Center, Albert Einstein." In *New Ways of Making Babies: The Case of Egg Donation*, edited by Cynthia B. Cohen, 15–28. Bloomington: Indiana University Press, 1996.

Barry, Brian. *Culture and Equality: An Egalitarian Critique of Multiculturalism.* Cambridge: Polity, 2001.

Bartholet, Elizabeth. *Family Bonds: Adoption and the Politics of Parenting.* Boston: Houghton Mifflin, 1993.

Bayne, Tim. "Gamete Donation and Parental Responsibility." *Journal of Applied Philosophy* 20 (2003): 77–87.

Bayne, Tim, and Avery Kolers. "'Are You My Mommy?' On the Genetic Basis of Parenthood." *Journal of Applied Philosophy* 18 (2001): 273–285.

———. "Toward a Pluralist Account of Parenthood." *Bioethics* 17 (2003): 221–242.

Beauchamp, Tom L., and James F. Childress. *Principles of Biomedical Ethics.* 6th ed. New York: Oxford University Press, 2009.

Beckwith, Francis J. "Personal Bodily Rights, Abortion, and Unplugging the Violinist." *International Philosophical Quarterly* 32 (1992): 105–118.

Benatar, David. *Better Never to Have Been: The Harm of Coming into Existence.* Oxford: Oxford University Press, 2006.

———. "The Unbearable Lightness of Bringing into Being." *Journal of Applied Philosophy* 16 (1999): 173–180.

———. "Why It Is Better Never to Come into Existence." *American Philosophical Quarterly* 34 (1997): 345–355.

Bettelheim, Bruno. *A Good Enough Parent: A Book on Child-Rearing.* New York: Alfred A. Knopf, 1987.

Blum, Lawrence A. *Friendship, Altruism, and Morality.* London: Routledge, 1980.

Blustein, Jeffrey. "Doing the Best for One's Child: Satisficing Versus Optimizing Parentalism." *Theoretical Medicine and Bioethics* 33 (2012): 199–205.

———. *Parents and Children: The Ethics of the Family.* New York: Oxford University Press, 1982.

———. "Procreation and Parental Responsibility." *Journal of Social Philosophy* 28 (1997): 79–86.

Boonin, David. "Better to Be." *South African Journal of Philosophy* 31 (2012): 10–25.

———. *A Defense of Abortion.* Cambridge: Cambridge University Press, 2002.

———. "A Defense of 'A Defense of Abortion': On the Responsibility Objection to Thomson's Argument." *Ethics* 107 (1997): 286–313.

Boswell, John. *The Kindness of Strangers: The Abandonment of Children in Western Europe from Late Antiquity through the Renaissance.* New York: Pantheon, 1988.

Brake, Elizabeth. "Fatherhood and Child Support: Do Men Have a Right to Choose?" *Journal of Applied Philosophy* 22 (2005): 55–73.

———. "Willing Parents: A Voluntarist Account of Parental Role Obligations." In *Procreation and Parenthood: The Ethics of Bearing and Rearing Children,* edited by David Archard and David Benatar, 151–177. Oxford: Oxford University Press, 2010.

Brakman, Sarah-Vaughan, and Sally J. Scholz. "Adoption, ART, and a Re-conception of the Maternal Body: Toward Embodied Maternity." *Hypatia* 21 (2006): 54–73.

Brennan, Samantha, and Robert Noggle. "The Moral Status of Children: Children's Rights, Parents' Rights, and Family Justice." *Social Theory and Practice* 23 (1997): 1–26.

Bridge, Andrew. *Hope's Boy.* New York: Hyperion, 2008.

Brighouse, Harry. "Civic Education and Liberal Legitimacy." *Ethics* 108 (1998): 719–745.

Brock, Dan W. "Is Selection of Children Wrong?" In *Human Enhancement,* edited by Julian Savulescu and Nick Bostrom, 251–276. Oxford: Oxford University Press, 2009.

Brodzinsky, David M. "A Stress and Coping Model of Adoption Adjustment." In *The Psychology of Adoption*, edited by David M. Brodzinsky and Marshall M. Schechter, 3–24. New York: Oxford University Press, 1990.

Brooks, David. "The Opportunity Gap." *New York Times*, July 10, 2012, sec. A.

———. "When Families Fail." *New York Times*, February 14, 2013, sec. A.

Brown, Douglas. "Good Practice for a Tough Fatherhood." *New York Times*, June 21, 2009, www.nytimes.com/2009/06/21/fashion/21love.html.

Brown, Harriet. "A Family Label, Ungarbled." *New York Times*, February 28, 2010, www.nytimes.com/2010/02/28/fashion/28love.html.

Broyde, Michael J. "Adoption, Personal Status, and Jewish Law." In *The Morality of Adoption: Socio-Psychological, Theological, and Legal Perspectives*, edited by Timothy P. Jackson, 128–147. Grand Rapids, Mich.: Eerdmans, 2005.

Buchanan, Allen. "Enhancement and the Ethics of Development." *Kennedy Institute of Ethics Journal* 18/1 (2008): 1–34.

Buchanan, Allen, Dan W. Brock, Norman Daniels, and Daniel Wikler. *From Chance to Choice: Genetics and Justice*. Cambridge: Cambridge University Press, 2000.

Burtt, Shelley. "In Defense of *Yoder*: Parental Authority and the Public Schools." In *Political Order: Nomos XXXVIII*, edited by Ian Shapiro and Russell Hardin, 412–437. New York: New York University Press, 1996.

———. "Religious Parents, Secular Schools: A Liberal Defense of an Illiberal Education." *The Review of Politics* 56 (1994): 51–70.

———. "Reproductive Responsibilities: Rethinking the Fetal Rights Debate." *Policy Sciences* 27 (1994): 179–196.

———. "Which Babies? Dilemmas of Genetic Testing." *Tikkun* 16/1 (2001): 45–47.

Cahill, Lisa Sowle. "Abortion and Argument by Analogy." *Horizons* 9 (1982): 271–287.

———. "Moral Concerns about Institutionalized Gamete Donation." In *New Ways of Making Babies: The Case of Egg Donation*, edited by Cynthia B. Cohen, 70–87. Bloomington: Indiana University Press, 1996.

Cahn, Naomi R., and Joan Heifetz Hollinger. *Families by Law: An Adoption Reader*. New York: New York University Press, 2004.

Callahan, Daniel. "Bioethics and Fatherhood." *Utah Law Review* 3 (1992): 735–746.

Callan, Eamonn. "Autonomy, Child-Rearing, and Good Lives." In *The Moral and Political Status of Children*, edited by David Archard and Colin Macleod, 118–141. Oxford: Oxford University Press, 2002.

Chambers, David L. "The Coming Curtailment of Compulsory Child Support." *Michigan Law Review* 80 (1982): 1614–1634.

———. "Fathers, the Welfare System, and the Virtues and Perils of Child-Support Enforcement." *Virginia Law Review* 81 (1995): 2575–2605.

Cohen, Cynthia B. "Parents Anonymous." In *New Ways of Making Babies: The Case of Egg Donation*, edited by Cynthia B. Cohen, 88–105. Bloomington: Indiana University Press, 1996.

Cohen, I. Glenn. "The Constitution and the Rights Not to Procreate." *Stanford Law Review* 60 (2008): 1135–1196.

———. "The Right Not to Be a Genetic Parent?" *Southern California Law Review* 81 (2008): 1115–1196.

Coontz, Stephanie. "The Evolution of American Families." In *Families as They Really Are*, edited by Barbara J. Risman, 30–47. New York: W.W. Norton, 2010.

———. *The Social Origins of Private Life: A History of American Families 1600–1900*. London: Verso, 1988.

Crenson, Matthew A. *Building the Invisible Orphanage: A Prehistory of the American Welfare System*. Cambridge, Mass.: Harvard University Press, 1998.

Daniels, Ken. "The Semen Providers." In *Donor Insemination: International Social Science Perspectives*, edited by Ken Daniels and Erica Haimes, 76–104. Cambridge: Cambridge University Press, 1998.

Daniels, Norman. *Am I My Parents' Keeper? An Essay on Justice between the Young and the Old*. Oxford: Oxford University Press, 1988.

———. "Duty to Treat or Right to Refuse?" *Hastings Center Report* 21/2 (1991): 36–46.

Davis, Dena S. "Genetic Dilemmas and the Child's Right to an Open Future." *Hastings Center Report* 27/2 (1997): 7–15.

Davis, N. Ann. "Fiddling Second: Reflections on 'A Defense of Abortion.'" In *Fact and Value: Essays on Ethics and Metaphysics for Judith Jarvis Thomson*, edited by Alex Byrne, Robert Stalnaker, and Ralph Wedgwood, 81–96. Cambridge, Mass.: The MIT Press, 2001.

DeGrazia, David. *Human Identity and Bioethics*. Cambridge: Cambridge University Press, 2005.

Donagan, Alan. *The Theory of Morality*. Chicago: The University of Chicago Press, 1977.

Edyvane, Derek. "Against Unconditional Love." *Journal of Applied Philosophy* 20 (2003): 59–75.

Elshtain, Jean Bethke. "The Chosen Family." *The New Republic*, September 14 and 21, 1998, 45–54.

English, Jane. "What Do Grown Children Owe Their Parents?" In *Having Children: Philosophical and Legal Reflections on Parenthood*, edited by Onora O'Neill and William Ruddick, 351–356. New York: Oxford University Press, 1979.

Erikson, Erik. *Identity: Youth and Crisis*. New York: W.W. Norton, 1968.

Feinberg, Joel. *Freedom and Fulfillment: Philosophical Essays*. Princeton: Princeton University Press, 1992.

Filmer, Robert. *Patriarcha and Other Writings*, edited by Johann P. Immerville. Cambridge: Cambridge University Press, 1991.

Fishkin, James. *Justice, Equal Opportunity, and the Family*. New Haven: Yale University Press, 1983.

Foot, Philippa. *Moral Dilemmas and Other Topics in Moral Philosophy*. Oxford: Oxford University Press, 2002.

———. *Virtues and Vices and Other Essays in Moral Philosophy*. Berkeley: University of California Press, 1978.

Fried, Charles. *Order and Law: Arguing the Reagan Revolution—A Firsthand Account*. New York: Simon & Schuster, 1991.

Friedman, Marilyn. *What Are Friends For? Feminist Perspectives on Personal Relationships and Moral Theory*. Ithaca, N.Y.: Cornell University Press, 1993.

Friedman, Richard A. "Accepting That Good Parents May Plant Bad Seeds." *New York Times*, July 12, 2010, sec. D.

Funke, Michael. "Fostering Independence: State Responsibility for Emancipated Youth." Unpublished.

Fuscaldo, Giuliana. "Genetic Ties: Are They Morally Binding?" *Bioethics* 20 (2006): 64–76.

Galston, William A. "Two Concepts of Liberalism." *Ethics* 105 (1995): 516–534.

General Court of Massachusetts. "An Act to Provide for the Adoption of Children (1851)." In *Families by Law: An Adoption Reader*, edited by Naomi R. Cahn and Joan Heifetz Hollinger, 9–10. New York: New York University Press, 2004.

George, Rolf. "On the External Benefits of Children." In *Kindred Matters: Rethinking the Philosophy of the Family*, edited by Diana Tietjens Meyers, Kenneth Kipnis, and Cornelius F. Murphy, Jr., 209–217. Ithaca, N.Y.: Cornell University Press, 1993.

———. "Who Should Bear the Cost of Children?" *Public Affairs Quarterly* 1 (1987): 1–42.

Gibbs, Nancy. "A Man's Right To Choose?" *Time*, March 15, 2006, www.time.com/ time/nation/article/0,8599,1173414,00.html.

Gilbert, Scott F. "When 'Personhood' Begins in the Embryo: Avoiding a Syllabus of Errors." *Birth Defects Research* 84/Part C (2008): 164–173.

Glover, Jonathan. *Choosing Children: Genes, Disability, and Design.* Oxford: Oxford University Press, 2006.

Griffiths, A. Phillips. "Child Adoption and Identity." In *Philosophy and Practice*, edited by A. Phillips Griffiths, 275–285. Cambridge: Cambridge University Press, 1985.

Gutmann, Amy. "Children, Paternalism, and Education: A Liberal Argument." *Philosophy and Public Affairs* 9 (1980): 338–358.

———. "Civic Education and Diversity." *Ethics* 10 (1995): 557–579.

Hansen, Drew D. "The American Invention of Child Support: Dependency and Punishment in Early American Child Support Law." *Yale Law Journal* 108 (1999): 1123–1153.

Hardimon, Michael O. "Role Obligations." *The Journal of Philosophy* 91 (1994): 333–363.

Harman, Elizabeth. "Critical Study." *Noûs* 43 (2009): 776–785.

Harris, George. "Fathers and Fetuses." *Ethics* 96 (1986): 594–603.

Harris, John. *Enhancing Evolution: The Ethical Case for Making Better People.* Princeton: Princeton University Press, 2007.

Hart, H. L. A. *The Concept of Law.* Oxford: Oxford University Press, 1961.

Held, Virginia. *Feminist Morality: Transforming Culture, Society, and Politics.* Chicago: The University of Chicago Press, 1993.

Henig, Robin Marantz. *Pandora's Baby: How the First Test Tube Babies Sparked the Reproductive Revolution.* Boston: Houghton Mifflin, 2004.

Henley, Kenneth. "The Authority to Educate." In *Having Children: Philosophical and Legal Reflections on Parenthood*, edited by Onora O'Neill and William Ruddick, 254–264. New York: Oxford University Press, 1979.

Heydt, Colin. "Practical Ethics in Eighteenth-Century Britain." In *The Oxford Handbook of Eighteenth-Century British Philosophy*, edited by James Harris, 369–389. Oxford: Oxford University Press, 2013.

Hobbes, Thomas. *Leviathan.* Edited by Edwin Curley. Indianapolis: Hackett, 1994.

Holland, Suzanne. "Contested Commodities at Both Ends of Life: Buying and Selling Gametes, Embryos, and Body Tissues." *Kennedy Institute of Ethics Journal* 11 (2001): 263–284.

Hostetler, John A. *Writing the Amish: The Worlds of John A. Hostetler.* Edited by David L. Weaver-Zercher. University Park: The Pennsylvania State University Press, 2004.

Hume, David. *A Treatise of Human Nature.* Edited by P. H. Nidditch, 2nd ed. Oxford: Oxford University Press, 1978.

Hursthouse, Rosalind. "Virtue Theory and Abortion." *Philosophy and Public Affairs* 20 (1991): 223–246.

Ivanhoe, Philip J. "Filial Piety as a Virtue." In *Working Virtue: Virtue Ethics and Contemporary Moral Problems*, edited by Rebecca L. Walker and Philip J. Ivanhoe, 297–312. Oxford: Oxford University Press, 2007.

Jeske, Diane. "Families, Friends, and Special Obligations." *Canadian Journal of Philosophy* 28 (1998): 527–556.

Johnson-Weiner, Karen M. *Train Up a Child: Old Order and Amish and Mennonite Schools.* Baltimore: The Johns Hopkins University Press, 2007.

Jones, Howard, Ian Cooke, Roger Kempers, Peter Brinsden, and Doug Saunders, ed. IFFS Surveillance 2010, www.iffs-reproduction.org/documents/IFFS_Surveillance_2010.pdf.

Kaczor, Christopher. *The Ethics of Abortion: Women's Rights, Human Life, and the Question of Justice*. Routledge: New York, 2011.

Kamm, Frances. "What Is and Is Not Wrong with Enhancement." In *Human Enhancement*, edited by Julian Savulescu and Nick Bostrom, 91–130. Oxford: Oxford University Press, 2009.

Kant, Immanuel. *Critique of Practical Reason*. Translated by Mary Gregor. Cambridge: Cambridge University Press, 1997.

———. *Critique of Pure Reason*. Translated by Norman Kemp Smith. New York: St. Martin's Press, 1929.

———. *Groundwork of the Metaphysics of Morals*. Translated by Mary Gregor. Cambridge: Cambridge University Press, 1997.

———. *Grundlegung zur Metaphysik der Sitten*. Edited by Karl Vorländer. 3rd ed. Hamburg: Felix Meiner, 1965.

———. *Kritik der praktischen Vernunft*. Edited by Horst D. Brandt and Heiner F. Klemme. Hamburg: Felix Meiner, 2003.

———. *Kritik der reinen Vernunft*. Edited by Raymund Schmidt. 3rd ed. Hamburg: Felix Meiner, 1990.

———. *The Metaphysics of Morals*. Translated by Mary Gregor. Cambridge: Cambridge University Press, 1998.

———. *Metaphysik der Sitten*. Edited by Karl Vorländer. 4th ed. Hamburg: Felix Meiner, 1966.

———. *Perpetual Peace and Other Essays*. Translated by Ted Humphrey. Indianapolis: Hackett, 1983.

———. *Werke. Schriften von 1783–1788*. Edited by Artur Buchenau and Ernst Cassirer. Vol. 4. Berlin: Bruno Cassirer, 1922.

Kass, Leon R. *Life, Liberty and the Defense of Dignity: The Challenge for Bioethics*. San Francisco: Encounter, 2002.

———. *Toward a More Natural Science: Biology and Human Affairs*. New York: The Free Press, 1985.

Keller, Simon. *The Limits of Loyalty*. Cambridge: Cambridge University Press, 2007.

Kolodny, Niko. "Which Relationships Justify Partiality? The Case of Parents and Children." *Philosophy and Public Affairs* 38 (2010): 37–75.

Korsgaard, Christine. *Creating the Kingdom of Ends*. Cambridge: Cambridge University Press, 1996.

Kraybill, Donald B. *The Riddle of Amish Culture*. Baltimore: The Johns Hopkins University Press, 1989.

Krimmel, Herbert T. "The Case against Surrogate Parenting." *Hastings Center Report* 13/5 (1983): 35–39.

———. "Surrogate Mother Arrangements from the Perspective of the Child." *Logos* 9 (1988): 97–112.

Kuczynski, Alex. "Her Body, My Baby." *New York Times Magazine*, November 30, 2008, 42ff.

Kunz, Diane B., Arthur Caplan, Charles P. Kindregan, Jr., and Rebecca Dresser. "The Baby Market." *New York Times*, December 29, 2009, http://roomfordebate.blogs.nytimes.com/2009/12/29/the-baby-market/.

Kupfer, Joseph. "Can Parents and Children Be Friends?" *American Philosophical Quarterly* 27 (1990): 15–26.

LaFollette, Hugh. "Licensing Parents." *Philosophy and Public Affairs* 9 (1980): 182–197.

Lang, Susan S. *Women without Children: The Reasons, the Rewards, the Regrets*. New York: Pharos Books, 1991.

Larkin, Philip. *Collected Poems*. Edited by Anthony Thwaite. New York: Farrar, Straus and Giroux, 2003.

Lauritzen, Paul. *Pursuing Parenthood: Ethical Issues in Assisted Reproduction*. Bloomington: Indiana University Press, 1993.

Levine, Aaron D. "Self-Regulation, Compensation, and the Ethical Recruitment of Oocyte Donors." *Hastings Center Report* 40/2 (2010): 25–36.

Lewontin, Richard. *The Triple Helix: Gene, Organism, and Environment.* Cambridge, Mass.: Harvard University Press, 2000.

Liao, S. Matthew. "The Idea of a Duty to Love." *The Journal of Value Inquiry* 40 (2006): 1–22.

———. "The Right of Children to Be Loved." *The Journal of Political Philosophy* 14 (2006): 420–440.

Lifton, Betty Jean. "Shared Identity Issues for Adoptees." In *Clinical and Practical Issues in Adoption: Bridging the Gap between Adoptees Placed as Infants and as Older Children,* edited by Victor Groza and Karen F. Rosenberg, 37–48. Westport, Conn.: Praeger, 1998.

Locke, John. *Two Treatises of Government.* Edited by Peter Laslett. Cambridge: Cambridge University Press, 1988.

MacIntyre, Alasdair. *Dependent Rational Animals: Why Human Beings Need the Virtues.* Chicago: Open Court, 1999.

Macleod, Colin. "Parental Responsibilities in an Unjust World." In *Procreation and Parenthood: The Ethics of Bearing and Rearing Children,* edited by David Archard and David Benatar, 128–150. Oxford: Oxford University Press, 2010.

Mahowald, Mary B. "Relinquishment and Adoption: Are They Genuine Options?" *Cambridge Quarterly of Healthcare Ethics* 5 (1996): 437–439.

Maienschein, Jane. *Whose View of Life? Embryos, Cloning and Stem Cells.* Cambridge, Mass.: Harvard University Press, 2003.

Malm, Heidi. "Paid Surrogacy: Arguments and Responses." *Public Affairs Quarterly* 3 (1989): 57–64.

Malmqvist, Erik. "Reprogenetics and the 'Parents Have Always Done It' Argument." *Hastings Center Report* 41/1 (2011): 43–49.

Marquardt, Elizabeth, Norval D. Glenn, and Karen Clark. *My Daddy's Name Is Donor: A New Study of Young Adults Conceived through Sperm Donation.* New York: Institute for American Values, 2010.

McCormick, Richard A. "Ambiguity in Moral Choice." In *Doing Evil to Achieve Good: Moral Choice in Conflict Situations,* edited by Richard A. McCormick and Paul Ramsey, 7–53. Chicago: Loyola University Press, 1978.

———. "Vive la Différence! Killing and Allowing to Die." *America,* December 6, 1997, 6–12.

McMahan, Jeff. *The Ethics of Killing: Problems at the Margins of Life.* Oxford: Oxford University Press, 2002.

———. "Wrongful Life: Paradoxes in the Morality of Causing People to Exist." In *Rational Commitment and Social Justice: Essays for Gregory Kavka,* edited by Jules L. Coleman and Christopher W. Morris, 208–247. Cambridge: Cambridge University Press, 1998.

Meyers, Thomas J. "Education and Schooling." In *The Amish and the State,* edited by Donald B. Kraybill, 86–106. Baltimore: The Johns Hopkins University Press, 1993.

Miller, Richard W. *Globalizing Justice: The Ethics of Poverty and Power.* Oxford: Oxford University Press, 2010.

Mills, Claudia. "The Child's Right to an Open Future?" *Journal of Social Philosophy* 34 (2003): 499–509.

———. "Duties to Aging Parents." In *Care of the Aged,* edited by James M. Humber and Robert F. Almeder, 147–166. Totawa, N.J.: Humana Press, 2003.

Millum, Joseph. "How Do We Acquire Parental Obligations?" *Social Theory and Practice* 34 (2008): 71–93.

———. Review of *Conceptions of Parenthood: Ethics and the Family,* by Michael W. Austin. *Notre Dame Philosophical Reviews,* April 26, 2008, http://ndpr .nd.edu/review.cfm?id=12946.

Milton, John. *The Complete Poetical Works of John Milton.* New York: Thomas Y. Crowell, 1892.

Miner, Robert. *Thomas Aquinas on the Passions: A Study of* Summa Theologiae *Ia2ae 22–48.* Cambridge: Cambridge University Press, 2009.

Montale, Eugenio. *Collected Poems 1920–1954.* Translated by Jonathan Galassi. Bilingual ed. New York: Farrar, Straus and Giroux, 1998.

Morgan, Jeffrey. "Children's Rights and the Parental Authority to Instill a Specific Value System." *Essays in Philosophy* 7/1 (2006), http://commons.pacificu.edu/cgi/viewcontent.cgi?article=1226&context=eip.

Murray, Thomas H. "New Reproductive Technologies and the Family." In *New Ways of Making Babies: The Case of Egg Donation,* edited by Cynthia B. Cohen, 51–69. Bloomington: Indiana University Press, 1996.

Nagel, Thomas. "Death." *Noûs* 4 (1970): 73–80.

Nelson, James Lindemann. "Genetic Narratives: Biology, Stories, and the Definition of the Family." *Health Matrix* 2 (1992): 71–83.

———. "Parental Obligations and the Ethics of Surrogacy: A Causal Perspective." *Public Affairs Quarterly* 5 (1991): 49–61.

Nietzsche, Friedrich. *The Birth of Tragedy.* Translated by Walter Kaufmann. New York: Random House, 1967.

———. *Die Geburt der Tragödie.* Stuttgart: Philipp Reclam, 1993.

Noggle, Robert. "Special Agents: Children's Autonomy and Parental Authority." In *The Moral and Political Status of Children,* edited by David Archard and Colin Macleod, 97–117. Oxford: Oxford University Press, 2002.

Nolan, Mark A., and Diana M. Grace. "Should Adopted Children Be Granted Access to the Identity of Their Birth Parents? A Psychological Perspective." *Journal of Information Ethics* 12 (2003): 67–79.

Nozick, Robert. *Anarchy, State, and Utopia.* New York: Basic Books, 1974.

O'Donovan, Oliver. *Begotten or Made?* Oxford: Oxford University Press, 1984.

Okin, Susan Moller. *Women in Western Political Thought.* Princeton: Princeton University Press, 1979.

O'Neill, Onora. "Begetting, Rearing, and Bearing." In *Having Children: Philosophical and Legal Reflections on Parenthood,* edited by Onora O'Neill and William Ruddick, 25–38. New York: Oxford University Press, 1979.

———. "Children's Rights and Children's Lives." *Ethics* 98 (1988): 445–463.

———. *Constructions of Reason: Explorations of Kant's Practical Philosophy.* Cambridge: Cambridge University Press, 1989.

———. "Ending World Hunger." In *Matters of Life and Death: New Introductory Essays in Moral Philosophy,* edited by Tom Regan, 235–279. 3rd ed. New York: McGraw-Hill, 1993.

———. "The 'Good Enough' Parent in the Age of the New Reproductive Technologies." In *The Ethics of Genetics in Human Procreation,* edited by Hille Haker and Deryck Beyleveld, 33–48. Aldershot: Ashgate, 2000.

———. *Towards Justice and Virtue: A Constructive Account of Practical Reasoning.* Cambridge: Cambridge University Press, 1996.

Overall, Christine. *Why Have Children? The Ethical Debate.* Cambridge, Mass.: The MIT Press, 2012.

Padawer, Ruth. "Losing Fatherhood." *New York Times Magazine,* November 22, 2009, 38ff.

Page, Edgar. "Donation, Surrogacy and Adoption." *Journal of Applied Philosophy* 2 (1985): 161–167.

Parfit, Derek. *Reasons and Persons.* Oxford: Oxford University Press, 1984.

Parker, Michael. "An Ordinary Chance of a Desirable Existence." In *Procreation and Parenthood: The Ethics of Bearing and Rearing Children,* edited by David Archard and David Benatar, 57–77. Oxford: Oxford University Press, 2010.

Paul, Annie Murphy. *Origins: How the Nine Months before Birth Shape the Rest of Our Lives*. New York: Free Press, 2010.

Pavlischek, Keith J. "Abortion Logic and Paternal Responsibilities: One More Look at Judith Thomson's 'A Defense of Abortion.'" *Public Affairs Quarterly* 7 (1993): 341–361.

Plato. *The Republic*. Translated by Allan Bloom. 2nd ed. New York: Basic Books, 1968.

Polgreen, Lydia. "Overcoming Customs and Stigma, Sudan Gives Orphans a Lifeline." *New York Times*, April 5, 2008, sec. A

Pollitt, Katha. "The Strange Case of Baby M." *The Nation*, May 23, 1987, www .thenation.com/article/strange-case-baby-m.

Presser, Stephen B. "The Historical Background of the American Law of Adoption." *Journal of Family Law* 11 (1972): 443–516.

Prewitt, Shauna R. "Giving Birth to a 'Rapist's Child': A Discussion and Analysis of the Limited Legal Protections Afforded to Women Who Become Mothers through Rape." *Georgetown Law Journal* 98 (2010): 827–862.

Prusak, Bernard G. "Double Effect, All Over Again: The Case of Sister Margaret McBride." *Theoretical Medicine and Bioethics* 32 (2011): 271–283.

———. "Rethinking 'Liberal Eugenics': Reflections and Questions on Habermas on Bioethics." *Hastings Center Report* 35/6 (2005): 31–42.

———. "A Riskier Discourse." *Commonweal*, November 23, 2012, 16–20.

Purdy, Laura. "Abortion and the Husband's Rights: A Reply to Wesley Teo." *Ethics* 86 (1976): 247–251.

———. "Surrogate Mothering: Exploitation or Empowerment?" *Bioethics* 3 (1989): 18–34.

Quinn, Warren. "Abortion: Identity and Loss." *Philosophy and Public Affairs* 13 (1984): 24–54.

Rachels, James. "Active and Passive Euthanasia." *New England Journal of Medicine* 292 (1975): 78–80.

Rawls, John. *Political Liberalism*. New York: Columbia University Press, 1996.

———. *A Theory of Justice*. Cambridge, Mass.: Harvard University Press, 1971.

Reeves, Philip. "Spread of 'Baby Boxes' Alarms Europeans." National Public Radio, February 18, 2013, www.npr.org/2013/02/18/172336348/spread-of-baby-boxes-alarms-europeans.

Rimm, Jennifer. "Booming Baby Business: Regulating Commercial Surrogacy in India." *University of Pennsylvania Journal of International Law* 30 (2008–2009): 1429–1462.

Robertson, John A. *Children of Choice: Freedom and the New Reproductive Technologies*. Princeton: Princeton University Press, 1994.

———. "Surrogate Mothers: Not So Novel After All." *Hastings Center Report* 13/5 (1983): 28–34.

Rosoff, Philip M. "The Myth of Genetic Enhancement." *Theoretical Medicine and Bioethics* 33 (2012): 163–178.

Ross, David. *The Right and the Good*. Edited by Philip Stratton-Lake. Oxford: Oxford University Press, 2002.

Roth, Philip. *The Human Stain*. New York: Random House, 2000.

Rothman, Barbara Katz. *The Tentative Pregnancy: Amniocentesis and the Sexual Politics of Motherhood*. New York: W.W. Norton, 1993.

Rousseau, Jean-Jacques. *Du contrat social ou Principes du droit politique*. Paris: Garnier Frères, 1962.

Sandel, Michael J. *The Case against Perfection*. Cambridge, Mass.: Harvard University Press, 2007.

———. "The Case against Perfection: What's Wrong with Designer Children, Bionic Athletes, and Genetic Engineering." *The Atlantic Monthly*, April 2004, 51ff.

———. "The Case against Perfection: What's Wrong with Designer Children, Bionic Athletes, and Genetic Engineering." In *Human Enhancement*, edited by Julian Savulescu and Nick Bostrom, 71–89. Oxford: Oxford University Press, 2009.

———. *Public Philosophy: Essays on Morality in Politics*. Cambridge, Mass.: Harvard University Press, 2005.

Satz, Debra. *Why Some Things Should Not Be for Sale: The Moral Limits of Markets*. Oxford: Oxford University Press, 2010.

Saul, Stephanie. "Building a Baby, with Few Ground Rules." *New York Times*, December 13, 2009, sec. A.

Savulescu, Julian. "Procreative Beneficence: Why We Should Select the Best Children." *Bioethics* 15 (2001): 413–426.

Scanlon, T. M. *Moral Dimensions: Permissibility, Meaning, Blame*. Cambridge, Mass.: Harvard University Press, 2008.

———. *What We Owe to Each Other*. Cambridge, Mass.: Harvard University Press, 1998.

Scheffler, Samuel. "Relationships and Responsibilities." *Philosophy and Public Affairs* 26 (1997): 189–209.

Schoeman, Ferdinand. "Rights of Children, Rights of Parents, and the Moral Basis of the Family." *Ethics* 91 (1980): 6–19.

Schrag, Francis. "Justice and the Family." *Inquiry* 19 (1976): 193–208.

Schwartz, Barry. *The Paradox of Choice: Why More Is Less*. New York: Harper-Collins, 2004.

Seabrook, John. "The Last Babylift: Adopting a Child in Haiti." *The New Yorker*, May 10, 2010, 44–53.

Shanley, Mary L. "Fathers' Rights, Mothers' Wrongs? Reflections on Unwed Fathers' Rights and Sex Equality." *Hypatia* 10 (1995): 74–103.

Shelley, Mary. *Frankenstein*. Edited by J. Paul Hunter. New York: W.W. Norton, 1996.

Shiffrin, Seana Valentine. "Wrongful Life, Procreative Responsibility, and the Significance of Harm." *Legal Theory* 5 (1999): 117–148.

Silverstein, Harry S. "On a Woman's 'Responsibility' for the Fetus." *Social Theory and Practice* 13 (1987): 103–119.

Simmons, A. John. "External Justifications and Institutional Roles." *Journal of Philosophy* 93 (1996): 28–36.

Spaemann, Robert. *Persons: The Difference between 'Someone' and 'Something.'* Translated by Oliver O'Donovan. Oxford: Oxford University Press, 2006.

Sparrow, Robert. "A Not-So-New Eugenics: Harris and Savulescu on Human Enhancement." *Hastings Center Report* 41/1 (2011): 32–42.

Sullivan, Ronald. "Sperm Mix-Up Lawsuit Is Settled." *New York Times*, August 1, 1991, sec. A.

"Surrogate Motherhood." ACOG Committee Opinion No. 397. *Obstetrics & Gynecology* 111 (2008): 465–470.

Thomson, Judith Jarvis. "A Defense of Abortion." *Philosophy and Public Affairs* 1 (1971): 47–66.

Triseliotis, John. "Identity Formation and the Adopted Person Revisited." In *The Dynamics of Adoption: Social and Personal Perspectives*, edited by Amal Treacher and Ilan Katz, 81–97. London: Jessica Kingsley, 2000.

Twain, Mark. *Huck Finn; Pudd'nhead Wilson; No. 44, The Mysterious Stranger; and Other Writings*. New York: Library of America, 2000.

Velleman, J. David. "Persons in Prospect." *Philosophy and Public Affairs* 36 (2008): 221–288.

Vischer, Robert. "All in the Family: When Should the State Intervene?" *Commonweal*, March 23, 2007, 8.

Walzer, Michael. *Exodus and Revolution*. New York: Basic Books, 1985.

Warner, Judith. "Outsourced Wombs." *New York Times*, January 3, 2008, http://opinionator.blogs.nytimes.com/2008/01/03/outsourced-wombs/.

Warnock, Mary. "'The Good of the Child.'" *Bioethics* 1 (1987): 141–155.

Warren, Mary Anne. "On the Moral and Legal Status of Abortion." *The Monist* 57 (1973): 43–61.

Wegar, Katarina. *Adoption, Identity, and Kinship: The Debate over Sealed Birth Records*. New Haven: Yale University Press, 1997.

Weinberg, Rivka. "Identifying and Dissolving the Non-Identity Problem." *Philosophical Studies* 137 (2008): 3–18.

———. "Is Having Children Always Wrong?" *South African Journal of Philosophy* 31 (2012): 26–37.

———. "The Moral Complexity of Sperm Donation." *Bioethics* 22 (2008): 166–178.

Wilkinson, Stephen. *Choosing Tomorrow's Children: The Ethics of Selective Reproduction*. Oxford: Oxford University Press, 2010.

Williams, Bernard. *Moral Luck: Philosophical Papers 1973–1980*. Cambridge: Cambridge University Press, 1981.

———. *Problems of the Self: Philosophical Papers 1956–1972*. Cambridge: Cambridge University Press, 1973.

Winnicott, D. W. *The Maturational Processes and the Facilitating Environment: Studies in the Theory of Emotional Development*. New York: International Universities Press, 1965.

Wittgenstein, Ludwig. *Philosophical Investigations*. Translated by G. E. M. Anscombe. 2nd, bilingual ed. Oxford: Basil Blackwell, 1958.

Wrobel, Gretchen Miller, Harold D. Grotevant, and Ruth G. McRoy. "Adolescent Search for Birthparents: Who Moves Forward?" *Journal of Adolescent Research* 19 (2004): 132–151.

Zelizer, Viviana A. *Pricing the Priceless Child: The Changing Social Value of Children*. Princeton: Princeton University Press, 1994.

Index

Printed and bound by CPI Group (UK) Ltd, Croydon, CR0 4YY

21/10/2024

01777082-0015